Abby Triebel

7/20

Cry Until You Laugh

Cry Until You Laugh

Real Love. Real Pain. Real Funny.

Kim Sorrelle

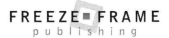
FREEZE FRAME publishing

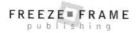

freezeframepublishing.com

Cry Until You Laugh
Copyright © 2012 Kim Sorrelle

Cover design by Amy Cole, JPL Design Solutions.

For more information on Kim Sorrelle, please visit
Web site: CryUntilYouLaugh.com
LinkedIn: Kim Sorrelle
Twitter: Kim Sorrelle
Blog and future book: datingat48.wordpress.com
Email: ksorrelle@gmail.com

Ms. Sorrelle is published in Tales of the Revolution: True Stories of People who are Poking the Box and Making a Difference by Seth Godin, 2011, The Domino Project, *Making a Difference in the Dominican Republic,*.

Library of Congress Control Number: 2012931754

ISBN 978-0-9839868-1-2

Dedication

This book is dedicated to
my dad, my first hero
and
my husband, my first love.

Acknowledgements

I love this page! I am so grateful that somebody way back when made the way for authors to acknowledge that no book could ever be written, no story could ever be told, no life could ever have meaning without the support, love, and encouragement of others.

My cousin Mary Jo Wesley worked her English teacher magic making my manuscript free of grammar, spelling and punctuation errors. She even made some very valuable suggestions leading me to try not to offend anyone. Thank you so much! (If anyone is offended by this book please email me and I will send it on to my cousin.)

My editor, now dear friend, Lorilee Craker spent hours poring over the pages, encouraging me every step of the way. I hope that we will continue to have lunch together at the local book store until death do us part. I highly recommend her editing and her writing. Google her, buy her books, hire her, you will be glad you did. Thank you so much to my marvelous looking girlfriend!

My publisher, Laura Hughes with Freeze Frame Publishing and Color House Graphics, is the reason that this book happened. Laura's homework, research and diligent efforts brought this baby home. Laura, I can never thank you enough, but I will give it my best shot. Thank you! And thank you for having such a wonderful sister, my best friend Sheila.

Doctors are not all the same. To find great doctors that you can talk to and trust is such an enormous blessing. I have been completely blessed by Dr. Ron Ford, Dr. Jamie Caughran, Dr. John LaGrand, Dr. Karen Dempsey, and Dr. Brett Brinker. Thank you for your kindness, patience, understanding and pulling all of those all-nighters to get your degrees. You are all the best. And you have some of the greatest staffs I have ever known.

Amanda, Paul, Luke, Noah and Cristian, thank you for being such awesome kids. Thank you for all of the help that you give me regularly. Thank you for giving me so many years of joy with so many more to come. Thank you for making Disney World our favorite place in the world. Thank you for being self-sufficient. Thank you for not breaking many bones or having many cavities when you were growing up. Thank you for staying out of jail. Thank you for trying to not embarrass me in public, I will try my hardest to return the favor. I love you!

Megan, Susie, Laci, and Sarah, thank you for loving my sons. Ray, thank you for loving my daughter. And thank you all for loving me. I love you tons!

My sister-in-law, LeeAnne, was at my house or me at hers nearly every day during the time that this book was written. LeeAnne, you are amazing. Thank you so much for everything. I would have lost my marbles long ago if not for you. Love you.

My sister-in-law, Andrea was there for me a ton and a call away always. Andi, thanks for great advice, great support and a great sense of humor. I am funnier than you are but you are pretty funny. Love you sis.

My mother-in-law turned mom, Nancy, is the best. Love you Mom.

Dad, you know you are my number one. Love you.

Mom, I have missed you for 21 years. I will never stop missing and loving you.

I have so many more that I need to thank so here is a blanket THANK YOU for the rest (you know who you are, yes, you).

Introduction

Just when I thought my life was planned out to the last wonderful detail, God sent someone who would turn my world upside down.

I never wanted to marry or (especially) bear children, and in my mind, I was on the fast track to becoming the first woman President of the United States. In school I started out with smiley faces that turned into A's & B's in later grades. I was near the top ten of my high school graduating class of '79 (Go Panthers!). My plan was to start down the presidential path by taking a Political Science Major at Michigan State University, followed by law school at George Washington University, with stints as a Senate Page and White House Intern thrown in the middle for good measure.

Then Steve walked into my life, and my visions of becoming President Kimberly Langlois faded quickly, replaced by new dreams.

I was nearing the end of my senior year in high school. I had dated plenty of guys, my chief aim for these dates being a fun dinner, a movie, and hopefully a great good night kiss. The last thing I was looking for was a potential husband.

I had casually met Steve the month before, by the pool table at Westgate Bowling Alley. At 6'3" to my almost 5'2", Steve had wavy brown hair, big brown eyes, and a "quietly confident" (another phrase for "stuck up") personality. He was a stud. When he called me to ask if I would come to his party, I acted coy for a minute. I told him I would have to check my calendar as I held my hand over the mouth piece of the phone, and jumped up and down for ten seconds. Some nerve, a guy calling on a Saturday morning for a party that night! I had to make him wait a little bit. After "checking my calendar," I happily accepted Steve's invitation then immediately called my first date for the evening and canceled.

That was May 5, 1979. Ten days later, I asked him to marry me while he was trying to steal kisses on my parents' couch. Less than a year later, on April 19, 1980, we were married, and by the next day I was ready to start a family (although we waited two years before having Amanda.)

Twenty eight years, five kids and five grandkids later, Steve still gave me butterflies in my stomach, and he still made my heart beat faster. I thought my perfect, happy life would go on forever, but my, my, how life can change in an instant.

ጸ ጸ ጸ

I was standing in my bathroom with two of my granddaughters in the bath tub, and my son, Noah, who was home from school for the weekend, when I got the call that would change everything. It was September 5, 2008, and for some reason I remember the exact time of day: 2:57 in the afternoon. The Surgical Oncologist's office called to tell me that the biopsy I had had two days prior was positive for breast cancer. The voice on the cordless phone was blathering on as I attempted to take notes on a pad of paper. "Blah, blah, blah, carcinoma, blah, blah, means cancer, blah… We will call you Tuesday with the next step, blah, blah…Don't worry. Try to have a nice weekend."

The crying started before I pushed "end" on the phone. Noah hugged me. I called Steve to tell him, but I could not stop wailing. He told me he was on his way home. I suppose it must have been Noah who helped the girls out of the bathtub. The moments immediately following that fateful call are a bit of a blur. I remember Steve finally getting home, and crying with me. He held me so tight, loved me so much. He apologized for anything he had ever done to hurt me. And we both cried out to God.

I knew I had to let my kids know immediately. And of course my dad had to be told, and Steve's mom, my brother's wife, who had kept Steve company during my biopsy, and my prayer warrior cousin Mary. Phone calls were made. People started arriving. Everyone was crying, except Noah, the rock of the family who rarely shows emotion.

Later in the evening someone was finally able to get a call through to my son, Luke. He, my daughter-in-law Megan, and their two kids had left just that morning to return to New York after two weeks of leave from the U.S. Navy.

I tried to act to tough. I heard the same words repeated all evening: *This is just a bump in the road, no big deal. Cancer research has come so far. Medicine in Grand Rapids has come a long way. Cancer is not like it used to be, it could be a lot worse. You are so strong. You will get through this. We're so sorry. What can I do to help? I will be there for you the whole way. I love you. I will pray for you.*

My brain was not processing much of it, even though my loved ones words were meant to encourage and soothe me. The phone call at 2:57 p.m. was the beginning of an out-of-body experience as I separated myself from the cancer diagnosis. It was so comforting to be surrounded by people that I loved, and loved me. Although I was physically present with my family and friends, I was somewhere else in my mind. Maybe that's why I didn't see how desperately Steve just needed to hold on to me for dear life.

When everyone was gone, Steve held me in bed all night long. Throughout the night I would wake up and cry some more, and Steve's arms would tighten around me. In the morning, I found out that my husband had not slept at all. This was totally unlike him. The man had slept through plenty of family Thanksgivings, and could sleep standing up if need be. Insomnia had never been an issue with Steve. If the Lions made a great play on a Sunday afternoon, I had to nudge him so he didn't miss it. I let him sleep through the Cowboys and Steelers, but never through overtime! By Monday morning, it seemed as if we had missed a whole week. Between the phone calls, crying, visitors, crying, football, and more crying, the weekend ended. It seemed to go on forever. I called my family doctor's office on Monday morning. They already had received a fax from the surgical oncologist with the biopsy results. The doctor was happy to prescribe sleeping pills and a little something for anxiety for both of us.

On Tuesday, I called to find out what to do next. I was told that the doctor wanted to do an MRI, which can take a couple of weeks to get scheduled. They had to obtain permission from my insurance company, and then find a time slot open for the one and only brand new, state of the art MRI machine in Grand Rapids. Thankfully—and surprisingly--my MRI was scheduled for the next day, Wednesday at 11:00 p.m. Waiting one day is much better than waiting for couple of weeks. I soon found out, however, that waiting is something that you have to get pretty good at as you go through a cancer diagnosis and treatment. I am practicing the art of waiting, and hopefully I am getting better at it each time I have to wait.

On that Friday, one week after hearing I had been diagnosed with breast cancer, the MRI results came in. I was with LeeAnne, my great friend, who also happens to be married to my brother (lucky man). We had lunch, and moved on to jewelry shopping when I received the phone call that would change my life. Again the words I heard came in dashes: *"Blah, blah, bad MRI, blah, this is tough news to give someone, blah, blah, really big on the left side, blah, blah, 9 centimeters by 3 centimeters, blah, blah, right side too, we think, blah, blah, blah, we will call you next Tuesday with the next step. Try to have a nice weekend."* At least this time I was able to hold the tears at bay until we were in the car.

My wonderful family and dear friends all wanted and needed to know news as it came. Keeping everyone posted on the twists and turns of my cancer journey seemed like an overwhelming challenge, so I decided to keep an email diary to keep my loved ones in the loop. What I didn't know then was how dramatic the bends in the road were to be. I didn't know I would suffer the profound loss of someone essential to me, just when I needed that person the most. My diary recorded every joy and tear, and is the basis for the book you hold in your hands today. Won't you join me as I travel through this rough terrain, and ultimately find a deeper grace than I thought possible?

And so it begins . . . .

September 15, 2008

After calling the surgical oncologist's office, I learned some bad news: the cancer is bigger than they expected, and there are growths on both sides of my breasts. The office is scheduling an MRI-guided biopsy for some time this week, and a mastectomy for sometime in the near future. They will be removing some lymph glands for testing.

Tomorrow, I am meeting with a surgeon at Lack's Cancer Center for a second opinion. On Thursday, I will be meeting with the rest of the team at Lack's, including a radiologist, oncologist, several nurses, etc. By the end of the week, Lack's will have their recommendation ready for a plan of action.

That's the medical update. I have to tell you, it's funny how life can change with a phone call. Everything was going along so well in my life when suddenly it was turned upside down.

On September 5, Steve and I looked forward to becoming empty nesters, as we would have the house to ourselves for the first time since Amanda was born in 1982. I was looking forward to quiet nights, line dancing again on Wednesday's with Cheri, cheaper utility bills, and a much smaller pile of laundry to deal with.

Instead, the phone rang.

With one phone call, quiet nights with a good book were transformed into researching, taking vitamins and praying instead.

Speaking of praying, here are some of my thoughts: I do believe in God. I do believe that God can heal anyone anytime because He is all powerful. I do believe that He knows that I have cancer because He is all-knowing. I do believe He cares, because He is Love. I do believe that I am not alone. I do believe that God will be with me in surgery, doctor's offices, and where ever I go. I do believe that God listens to our prayers so I will keep on talking to Him, and I hope that you will too.

I do not believe that He gave me cancer. I do not believe that there is a special thing to say or not say, or do or not do, so that God will heal me.

Mat Kearney wrote a great song called "Closer to Love." The lyrics resonate with me now more than ever. God is love. Getting closer to love is getting closer to God. I need to be praying every day that God pulls me "closer to love." After all, like the song says, I am someone who received the phone call that brought me to my knees, in more ways than one.

You, God, pull me closer to love.

God is good, all the time. All the time, God is good.

September 23, 2008

I finally received some good news: The results of the biopsy that I had done on my right side came back with no cancer! Praise God!

Today, I met with a wonderful plastic surgeon, Dr. Ford, and a great surgical oncologist, Dr. Caughran. Both doctors work out of Lack's Cancer Center in Grand Rapids. It seems I have two options:

1. Partial Mastectomy - I would undergo a Bracketed MRI where the Radiologist would put three or so wires in at the ends and middle of the cancer. Then Dr. Caughran

would remove the area along with margins and "Sentinel Glands," which are nodes or growths that "stand sentinel," or guard, over a nearby tumor. Provided that the margins and glands are all cancer free, I would then have radiation once a day for six and a half weeks.

2. Full Mastectomy - Dr. Caughran would perform the surgery, and Dr. Ford the reconstruction surgery all on the same day.

Either way, the cancer did test positive for "estrogen receptors," which means that estrogen is causing my tumor to grow, and the cancer should respond well to hormone suppression treatments. The plan is for me to meet with another oncologist who would then prescribe Tamoxifin. One Tamoxifin pill a day for five years is supposed to cut the chances of re-occurrence by 50%.

On Thursday afternoon, we are attending a multi-disciplinary clinic where Dr. Caughran, a radiologist, and an oncologist will all be there at the same time to review everything and make the final recommendations. Dr. Caughran had copies of everything, except the MRI that I had done two weeks ago, which she needs to see before making her final recommendations.

I could be having surgery as soon as next week Monday or Wednesday, if an MRI can be coordinated with surgery that soon, or Dr. Caughran and Dr. Ford can coordinate everything that soon.

I am praying that the cancer is contained, and not advancing anywhere else in my body.

I want you to know I am so grateful for your prayers and support. I feel God's presence, so thank you.

I believe God is not just one-dimensional, and/or impersonal. I believe God goes way beyond a being, sitting in Heaven, looking down, and marking us on our smart and stupid moves in a heavenly book. God wants us to know Him on a personal, conversational level, as his dear friend. So, I talk to God, and He talks back, and sometimes I am not too distracted to hear him.

I know God spoke to me in the middle of the night on August 27, 2008 (I had my first biopsy on September 3 and diagnosis on September 5). This is what He told me:

My child, listen to me. You will go through a trial, a time of mourning and sadness. But know that through it all I am by your side. At the end, true happiness will be found. Do not give up, do not despair. I will be with you always. It is okay, for you have been preparing for this time. Rest in Me. Trust in Me. Stay the course. Do not waiver, for those around you will look to you for strength, My strength. Let your light shine. I love you. My love is everlasting. Stay the course.

God is good. He is faithful to deliver all that He has promised. I thank God I do not need to rely on my own strength and wisdom. He provides both strength and wisdom, and so much more.

God is good; all the time.

September 26, 2008

I found out yesterday my options have been narrowed to one. The surgeon, after reviewing the MRI, said a full Mastectomy was my only choice because of the size of the mass. I hopefully will know the surgery date soon. Well, in the words of Solomon, "Vanity of vanity, all is vanity." There are plenty of people with cancer who wish it was as simple as cutting off a part of your body that you really don't need anyway.

I have to admit, even though 'they' are attached, I am really not all that attached to them. My biggest decision right now seems to be one breast or both breasts. I am looking into genetic testing to see if this was a gift from my ancestors, or if I just got lucky. If it is genetic, the chances of re-occurrence go up to about 50%. The other factor is that the Tamoxifin, which is necessary if you decide to keep one breast, would send me into the fabulous world of hot flashes and mood swings.

I am not ready to wear a red floppy hat with my purple leather dress! I know that menopause has to happen sooner or later, but I am enjoying my current disposition, and don't wish to become the Bride of Frankenstein. I have also seen too many of my gender fanning themselves outside their West Michigan homes in January. Then there are the husbands who have taken on life mantras like "Happy wife, Happy life," and those ever-repeated words "Yes dear." Poor Steve! This is all happening just when we were beginning to gain our independence together.

A couple of people in my immediate family would be more comfortable if I just bite the bullet and go with the two-for-one-special. "Why would you put new siding on just half of the house?" my son Paul said yesterday. Well put.
But I have a little bit of time to decide. One great advantage is they tattoo the center of your new, reconstructed breasts so I would get to pick the color. Hmm . . . the possibilities!

As I ponder my decision, please pray with me that I make the right one, and that I am sensitive to God's answers and wisdom and to my family. That the cancer is all contained and not invasive, and that the peace that now surrounds me is felt also by my husband, kids, and everyone else I know and love!

God is good, all the time.

P.S. Thank you for buying any product with the pink ribbons symbol! All of that research, funded by donations by food manufacturers etc, has led to great success in overcoming the body snatcher called "breast cancer."

October 1, 2008

Tomorrow morning, before the sun rises (in California, at least), Steve and I are flying to the state with the Big Apple. Our trip has nothing to do with my chest and everything to do with my sanity. My son, "Navy Nuke Luke," is in the last part of his training to be a Naval Nuclear Engineer in Saratoga Springs, New York. This is the locale where he, very unfairly, moved his wonderful wife and my beautiful and intelligent grandchildren. We are going for a long weekend while I can still go "intact."

Not much happened this week, medically speaking. I did go in today for all of the pre-surgery stuff (EEG, chest X-ray, blood work etc). I also had blood drawn for the genetic testing. Hopefully the results will be back before surgery.

I do not have a surgery date. I have found out that coordinating a surgical oncologist, a plastic surgeon, the right equipment, and a surgical ward is not as easy as one might think. Still, I'm pretty sure that my veterinarian brother used to neuter cats in the garage, so how hard can it all be, really? This is why you do not pray for patience. God will give it to you.

I haven't decided on the matter of one or two breasts yet. I am leaning toward having two removed for several reasons.

First, I do not want to go through this again. Second, my family would have more peace of mind, and third, I don't want to be always leaning to the right. Oh, and fourth, "The Change." Yes, I know, it's not that bad. You can wear summer clothes all year round. You don't roast chestnuts on an open fire anyway. Everyone already thinks you are a bit of a _____ (insert your own word here). *Blah, Blah, Blah*. It seems all of the men I know start to lose their hearing as their wives lose their girl-hood. Is this a coincidence or a blessing? You be the judge.

Please pray with me for wisdom, that the genetic testing comes back quickly, for surgery schedules to work out, and for my husband's sanity.

God bless you. God is good, all the time.

October 3, 2008

As everyone around the country gathers to celebrate National Apple Day, I will be having mine removed, my "apples," that is. The date has been set: October 21, National Apple Day as well as the 39th Birthday of Salman bin Hamad Bin Isa Al Dhalifa, crown prince of Bahrain. I hope he has a huge party.

I am looking forward to the surgery about as much as someone who deeply desires to get rid of a horrible toothache, but shivers when they think about the root canal that will relieve their pain. I am trying my best not to think about it, but everywhere I turn I see pink. Pink blenders, pink hats, pink pots, pink spatulas, pink bracelets, *pink everything*! On billboards, in store windows, on T.V.—it's all pink this month, also National Breast Cancer Awareness Month. There are even pink M & M's for goodness sake. It is great, don't misunderstand me. But just when I have forgotten about "NB Day" (NEW 'you know what' DAY), I turn around and there is a pink ribbon on something.

My options, as I see them, are to not leave my home, and screen all media for the next eighteen days, or look to the surgery with optimistic anticipation. I either hide from the world, or I try to figure out how to face this thing head on. I want to win. I like winning. I coached volleyball and basketball for years. I can tell you firsthand that losing stinks. The worst losses are those when you know you are better than the other team, yet somehow the scoreboard shows your opponent ahead at the end. Right now my opponent is cancer. Ha! I will defeat this adversary like every NFL team is taking it to the Detroit Lions this year.

Praise God I am not alone. God amazes me. I feel your prayers—the prayers of all my loved ones, friends, acquaintances and even strangers—as if they were arms wrapped around me in a kind, peaceful, loving embrace. I can feel the arms of God. Thank you.

God is good, all the time.

October 10, 2008

There are eleven more days until NB Day. It is an odd feeling, having an "alien" living in my body; one, if left to its own devises, could wreak havoc on my entire system. Eleven days must be just right because if not, then on day twelve my alien would burst out of my stomach, and begin attacking everyone in sight, just like in that old Sigourney Weaver movie, "Alien."

Over the years, while I have been dealing with a body weight not considered ideal on the American Medical Charts (even with

2" heels), I have daydreamed about the two situations through which I would surely and forever lose the weight.

The first is divorce. I have seen a lot of women transition from frumpy soccer mom to *Oo la la* lady, because their dreams of happily-ever-after came to a screeching halt. I thought if Steve would just leave me for a little while, I too could make that wonderful transformation, and he would beg me to take him back again. And, of course, we would live happily ever after. The problem is, I really love the guy and like to be with him. I think he likes me too because he never acts like the jerks that other women kick out of their houses. Plus, I have never had reason to call "Cheaters" to come and film an episode. So, my first idea for rapid weight loss has never materialized, and this has left me fat and sassy--and happily married.

My second weight loss idea was cancer. You know, a little chemo, a little sickness, nothing serious, just until my weight reaches 'Boy she looks great in a bikini.' Be careful what you wish for, right? I got cancer. No chemo yet and hopefully never. But, there is some weight loss. Before I knew I had cancer, I visited my family doctor to discuss my allergies. I had lost ten pounds in the four weeks since my last visit. She asked me how I did it. Of course, being the seasoned dieter and exercise enthusiast that I am, I told her that I was eating much healthier, and getting off the couch more often. She congratulated me, and said that she was glad that it was my efforts, and not some undetected cancer that was causing the weight loss. I have now lost twenty two pounds, and I cannot take any credit for losing the weight. I am on the high-antioxidant, no sugar, no flour, no potatoes, no rice, no bread, no fun diet. I am sure that helps, but I am not exercising at all; in fact, I'm on the couch more than ever. My head is optimistic, but my body feels like a vegetable, and not a healthy one that gives you lots of vitamins and minerals, and improves your eye sight to 20/20 vision. I feel like the kind of vegetable that does nothing but clog up your digestive system and seems to come out whole on the other end—ie: useless!

The other night I was sitting on the couch doing needle work with my reading glasses on! When did I turn into my grandmother? All I needed was deeper crow's feet, bad hearing, and a helmet hair-do, and you could have called me Dorothy or Florence. I loved my grandmothers, but I consider myself one of the cool Uma's (my grandbabies call me "Uma," like Uma Thurman, fitting, I thought, considering my coolness).

You know those cool grandmas, the ones that still shop at Express, wear boots that are made for walkin', and a hair style from an expensive salon in several colors, none of which God gave them. I am the hip Uma who decorates her house from Pier 1 instead of a cow and chicken motif; the one that travels to far away, exotic places to help people in need. Kind of like Uma Thurman, Martha Stewart and Mother Theresa rolled up in one, with a little Miley Cyrus thrown in just to bring down the average age. Hopefully I am just going through my slow crawling caterpillar phase, and will metamorphose to Umartesa Cyrus very soon. Watch out, world!

Thanks so much for all of the prayers and support. I know I would be going pretty nutty if you were not there for me. Your prayers keep my mind from focusing on NB Day. Your prayers keep my focus on the hand that is holding mine, my Lord.

God is good, all the time.

October 13, 2008

I decided to spend last night before NB in the hospital. Well, I didn't have much choice, as it turned out.

I had this bad, naughty pain in my chest that reached up my neck. I felt like I was way too deep in the ocean. It didn't last long, but long enough that they gave me a private room (suite, really, bathroom included!) in the heart area of Spectrum's Emergency Center. Several rounds of blood work, chest X-rays, and treadmill runs later, I found out a couple of very important things:

    1. Spectrum takes hearts very seriously.

    2. It is possible for me to get a bruise every time they draw blood.

    3.   I can smell pretty bad after just 10 minutes on a tread mill.

    4. God is good, all the time!

Number four is not some sort of secret, but sometimes I need to be reminded of it anyway. God showed up, as usual. I have had this little heart thing in the past. My heart skipped beats, and I have had a "lazy valve" that required taking antibiotics before seeing the dentist. I always hoped it wouldn't require surgery down the road.

Well, move over Kim and let God in! I found out that not only do I have the heart of a young, somewhat mysterious woman (I made that last part up), but all of my valves are great. That is right: No more lazy valves. And I don't think that it has anything to do with the fact that I read "Top Ten Habits of Very Hard Working People." I thank God I can go into surgery next week knowing my heart is right in more ways than one.

So, here we are, one week and one day until NB Day. What am I feeling? Peace that surpasses all understanding. Peace I can only attribute to your prayers. Thanks much.

My daughter-in-law suggested that next Monday, NB Day Eve, we celebrate the "OB's." I do not have to tell you which one of my sons' wives suggested this because, frankly, any one of them could have come up with the same idea. Her suggestion had something to do with flashing, which I think is illegal in Michigan, so don't expect to see me on "*Girls Gone Wild Grand Rapids.*" I do think I will celebrate in some way. Dinner at the Melting Pot sounds great. Anyone interested? Perhaps I'll do a little line dancing, if there is such a thing on Monday nights. Really, I would be happy to do anything to take my mind off of the next day.

Please keep those prayers coming!

God is good, all the time.

October 15, 2008

Several friends and family members have wondered what kind of fun event will take place on Monday night (NB Day Eve), so here it is. There is a little restaurant on Chicago Drive, in the thriving metropolis of downtown Grandville; it is creatively named "Chicago Drive Pub." We will be there from 6:00 p.m. on enjoying a last meal, sipping non-alcoholic Pina Coladas, and putting quarters in the juke box. Come one, come all! I plan on dancing my cares away, and do not want to be alone on the dance floor. Then I would look like some drugged out, self-absorbed freak, and that wouldn't be pretty. It should be a great time, and all-you-can-drink-ice water is on me!

My pre-surgery brochure dictates I must have no alcohol or recreational drugs within 24 hours of surgery. That is why my Pina Colada will be non-alcoholic. I guess that also means taking Mobic for my tennis elbow is out.

I have not heard back about the genetic testing. Please pray I hear really soon so I can give a final answer to whether I want to keep one breast or have both removed. I wonder if the doctor will ask me in a Regis Philbin-like voice if it truly is my final answer. Then I will have to pause, take a deep breath and say "Yes, doctor, that's my final answer." Then part of me will start flashing green, and the crowd will go wild! Oh, for the reassurance of making the right choice! Please pray also that part of me does not start flashing colors, but that God makes it really clear which way to go.

God is good, all the time. Thanks again and again. I hope to see you on Monday, October 20.

October 16, 2008

Good news! The cancer I have is *not* hereditary. Bad news: I blame the environment! Yes, you people who have polluted our lands, added preservatives to our foods, driven cars that emit toxic wastes, and sent your own waste into our water systems! You, who have super-sized, deep fried, and chocolate-covered everything we eat. You, the mega users have become mega polluters. You, who have operated factories and turned a blind eye to the smoke stacks. You, who filled our landfills with your excessive waste, and used more than three squares every time you wiped and therefore destroyed our rainforests!

Just kidding! It is not your fault, truly. Although, I must say, a few of the books I have read on cancer claim it *is* your fault. The other books I have read tell me it is my fault. Obviously, that cannot be true. Certainly my desire for black licorice, chips and dip, and chocolate is because those foods contain some nutritional value my body must be craving.

So, if it isn't your fault, and it isn't my fault, who do I blame? My theory is that when God created the world it was perfect. No pesticides or herbicides needed to be used. People could dig a hole in the back forty and cover it up after they did their business with no harm done to their surroundings. Trees produced beautiful, juicy fruit, plants yielded great vegetables, and the water was all potable. God created it all for us, and then gave it all to us with just one simple request about one simple tree. Then the whole thing happened with Eve and Adam (yes, Adam too) and the forbidden fruit. The next thing you know we have pesticides, war, and clothes.

God seems to be an easy target for blame. Hurricane Katrina was called God's vengeance on sinful New Orleans. An earthquake in San Francisco must be God's statement regarding homosexuality. An alcoholic gets liver disease because God does not approve of his drinking. A drug user dies of AIDS, the disease that God spewed on a sinful world filled with drug and sex abusers.

I say bologna.

I think after God gave us the earth and all it contains at the beginning of our human existence, we did what we did, and now every once in a while the earth burps, crops fail, rivers dry up, and someone we know gets cancer. This time it is my turn.

I have decided on the two-for-one breast removal deal. I guess Monday night I will have to do a double shot of green tea to celebrate. It took me this long to gain peace with a decision. It is not an easy one, but now I do feel that it is the right one, for me. I have read and heard so many things over the last seven weeks. What I know now is that everyone has to work this out for themselves. Everyone is different; every ride is different. For me it came down to selfishness. I do not want to wonder when or if my remaining breast would go haywire. I would love to be noble, and say it's for my family's peace of mind, but really it's for my peace of mind. Now, all I have to decide is the size, shape and color. Decisions, decisions, what is a woman to do? Thanks for the prayers. The timing of finding out the hereditary blood test results was perfect.

God is good, all the time.

October 19, 2008

A word of caution: This journal entry is going to be a bit 'R' rated, so get the kids out of the room, and cover your eyes during the bad parts. If you are not married, you need to stop reading at the end of paragraph four. If you are married, and do not know me that well, you might want to stop reading, too, otherwise we are going to be very close friends by the time your reading is done.

Today is significant. It is two days before NB Day. It is also the day that my Megan (Luke's wife) came into the world twenty three years ago. Happy Birthday Megan!

I am feeling very vulnerable today. Man, this whole breast cancer thing brings with it a lot of raw emotion. Friday, I cried because my doctor's office offered the viewing of an after-surgery patient because, in their words, *"it can be quite shocking."*

No kidding. I have seen flat chests before. My husband's chest is kind of flat, except for the bulging pectoral muscles. My kids have had flat chests at different times of their development. The guys that I had crushes on as a middle schooler in the 1970's had flat chests: David Cassidy, Michael Jackson, Davy Jones, Peter Brady, Little Joe, and Nick Barkley (everyone else liked Heath; I got Nick all to myself). I probably used to have a flat chest, too. I just don't remember it. I think that girls don't think about their chest until they begin to train it with a bra. My training started pretty early. I think I left my flat chest days back in 4th grade. In fact, I would have to say that I must have had a pretty darn good trainer because things seemed to turn out okay. The thing that I have not seen is a nipple-less flat chest. This thought hit me, and I cried: In a few short days my breasts were going to go from being a part of me to being dissected in a lab, and then thrown out with the evening trash. All of that training would end up in the Market Street Incinerator.

I cried again yesterday. Mostly, I cried because my cousin Beth was celebrating the wedding of her son Danny and new daughter-in-law Michele. I love them so much, and am so proud to have them in my life. I cried because I was too tired and exhausted to attend. I am sure that they had a great day. They were all so excited, and so was I. But, thanks cancer, "Wedding Kim," as Cousin Mary calls me, stayed home and watched Michigan State get their football behinds kicked, and Michigan beat Penn State in the first half. I love football but love my cousins more. I was wallowing in self-pity.

Today I cried again. Completely unexpectedly, tears and sobs came without any warning, kind of like those house guests that stop by in the middle of dinner, or worse, in the middle of a fight with your teenage daughter. Despite the bad timing, the tears came anyway.

Following a little afternoon delight with my beloved, (I warned you about the "R" rating), a stolen moment that seldom happens with kids and grandkids around, I cried like a baby and couldn't stop. Steve held me, and I held on like my life depended on it. My eyes are welling up just thinking about it so I apologize if the typing is a little fuzzy.

There we were, me crying, he telling me everything is going be okay, over and over, and over and over. Then it hit me. I knew why I was crying. I had just experienced my last roll in the hay completely intact. I showed up for the rendezvous in a sexy, lacy little something that I filled out quite nicely. As I lay there afterward, I knew I would never fill it out that way again. Nobody warned me that I would go from complete ecstasy to a complete mess in a matter of seconds. Where is all this information in those cancer books that have limited my diet and scared me with their scientific lingo? How about an emotional heads up as I approach the big day? And why, when I thought I felt so unattached to my breasts, am I suddenly so attached to the darn things that I wept over losing them?

If you have been reading my journal entries from the beginning, you might remember I had heard God tell me some things. One of those things was that I was going to have a time of mourning. As I shared that in an update, I did not know entirely what God was talking about. Some of it was obvious even way back on diagnosis day, September 5. But I figured parts of God's message to me I would discover later. This is one of them. *Mourning.* I am mourning the loss of my breasts. As a woman, who no longer has infant feeding in her future, it is easy to say "What do we need these things for?" or "I am sick of carrying them around everywhere I go." But in truth I think we do like them. It's part of what makes us a woman, part of our sexuality.

I am resting up for tomorrow night, my chest's last hurrah. I will be dancing the night away at Chicago Drive Pub. I hope you can come.

Thanks for the prayers and encouraging words. You are the best.

God is good, all the time.

October 21, 2008

NB Day!

Today is the day. My chest, both sides of it, will be leaving in a few minutes to walk the Green Mile. As they wheel me on the stretcher through the sterile hallways, I will surely get some sympathetic looks and understanding nods.

Although I am fairly certain that nervousness should enter my being soon, right now I have peace, the same peace that has surrounded me since the beginning of this adventure.

I will have surgery at St. Mary's Hospital, and then be wheeled over to Lack's Cancer Center for an as yet undetermined number of days. The Lacks people try to get you excited about your stay by telling you that there is a chef on the floor, and each patient orders from a menu. Yippy. A liquid diet prepared by a chef! *Mmmmm.* I can almost taste that beef broth now.

In less than an hour, I will transform from one of the walking free to a patient, an in-patient at that. It is an interesting word that hospitals and doctors use. I would prefer to be considered a guest. I surely do not want to overstay my welcome. You know what they say about guests and fish after three days. This way I will be sure to be home by the weekend.

Thanks so much for the party last night. It was a blast. I danced the night away. What a wonderful way to celebrate with family and friends. They did not have green tea, but I toasted all who were unable to attend with a great big glass of ice water. Thanks so much for all of you who did come. It is so comforting and reassuring to know that I am loved. Or was it the free food? Either way, my heart is warm.

Today more prayers will be answered. Thanks so much. Really!

God is good, all the time.

October 25, 2008

I am home. After three nights in a computerized, form-to-your-body hospital bed, with compassionate nurses giving around-the-clock attention, a full kitchen at my beck and call, beautiful flowers, a basket of heavenly green tea, some great books, and even greater friends and family as visitors, I am home.

Still, I would not recommend the surgery. I woke up in quite a bit of pain. The hourly doses of morphine made me loopy, but didn't take away my pain as much as I would have liked. I would, however, highly recommend the surgeons. Dr. Jamie Caughran, surgical oncologist, not only does incredible work, but has a bedside manner that would be closer on to Mother Theresa than Dr. House from TV's "House." Dr. Ford, my plastic surgeon, gave me a new chest right from the start.

My NB is not a completed work of art, but it is a good start. Dr. Ford told my waiting family and friends that I had impressive pectoral muscles, probably even bigger than his. This meant he had plenty of room to put some added saline in the expanders.

I am sure that I have Lynne and Alice to thank at the gym for all of those bench presses. Ahhh, another thing that I will not be doing for a long, long time! The nice people at pre-surgery put a few happy drugs into my I.V. so that I would not be anxious wheeling down to surgery. The last thing I remember is the anesthesiologist, also wonderful, placing a mask over my face, and telling me to go to my happy place. I started trying to figure out where my happy place is. Disney World? A warm beach with a cold Pina Colada? Ever since then I have been trying to decide where my happy place is. I think that today, my happy place is going to be at home, wrapped up in a warm blanket, lounging on the lazy boy, watching MSU give it to U of M. *Mmmmm*. That is a happy place. Someday my happy place will be heaven, but not today. Today it is Byron Center and Ann Arbor.

Thank you so much for the party on Monday night. I had a blast. What a great way for me and my two departing body parts to spend their last night out on the town. They really enjoyed it, and so did I. My brother Joel has offered to donate his nipples to me, and would like us to plan a going away party for them too. It is a very generous offer, but I have seen his hairy areolas and I am concerned about the maintenance. Maybe we should just have the party without the actual donation. I have seen Dr. Ford's work, and none of it has appeared hairy in the least. Plus, over the years Joel has had a certain pride in his upper half, and I would hate to be the one that hurts his Herculean looks in any way.

Our first batch of news has been very good. The initial reports on the sentinel glands did not show a spread of cancer-- yeah! The full pathology report will hopefully arrive at Dr. Caughran's office on Monday, so I should know a lot more then. Thanks for the prayers that our Great God is answering. Thank you Lord for the answers to all of those prayers.

God is good, all the time.

October 28, 2008

Today is the one week anniversary of my new chest, and I have great news! The pathology report showed no cancer on the right side, but several areas of cancer on the left. There was one area where they did not get enough margins, but they think they did get all of the cancer. Praise the Lord from whom all blessings flow!

I visited Dr. 90210 (a.k.a. Dr. Ford) today. I no longer have to pin those lovely drain bags onto my tee shirts. I was surprised how long they were. There must have been eighteen inches of tubing in each side. Starting next Thursday, the doctor will begin the plumping up process. I asked him about size, and he told me that one good thing about expanders is you can add to them, live with them for a while, and let some out or possibly add some more. I think that every woman who reads this should be a bit jealous. Can you imagine being able to flatten your chest a bit for a volleyball game then pump it up to fill out that new sweater? There has to be some money in this somewhere.

This week's plan of action is to relax and enjoy the warm fuzzy feelings that the pain meds give me. I am not allowed to do too much. Frankly, I do not feel like doing much. How often in life are you allowed to be lazy without it being a sin? I plan on taking full advantage of my slothfulness. I have a stack of books to read when my eyes are not too fuzzy from the valium, and of course there is all of that great stuff to watch on daytime television. I just hope that there is a good ten-step program if I end up addicted to TRU TV.

I have to tell you about the moment I saw my post-surgery chest. You know, that moment on the Lifetime Movies where the woman is in the bathroom, alone, after returning from her mastectomy. She stands there in a fluffy white robe, staring and waiting. Slowly she puts her hands up toward her neck feeling the plushness of the housecoat. Her hands move lower and find the belt that holds it all together. Carefully, she unties the slipknot, loosens the belt and opens up her covering. Her eyes never leave their reflection in the mirror. Then, when the robe is fully open her eyes begin to move down very slowly, first to her parched, pouty lips, then to her long, elegant neck, a little lower to the top of her chest, and then there it is! She sees her post-surgery body for the very first time. The perky grapefruits that used to fill that space are gone, replaced by lines of stitches. She struggles to wrap her mind around what she is seeing. Where did they go? She stares blankly as tears begin to well in her eyes. Oh, where did they go?

That was not my moment.

As I was being discharged from the hospital I found out that I could remove this beautiful vest bra that my insurance company is paying for and take a shower when I got home. Man, did that sound good. As soon as I arrived, Steve and I went right into the bathroom for the great unveiling. So, there I was in front of the mirror, wearing only the pretty vest and a pair of silky maroon striped undies (part of my intimate apparel had to be fun). First, Steve unzipped the vest, only to discover that there were a few hooks also holding it in place. He unhooked number one, then number two, but by the time he got to number three, the pain was intense I thought I was going to vomit and pass out. He rushed me over to the bed where I stayed sweating for quite some time. That's how my Lifetime Movie Moment went down. I guess that I was ready to see them, but they were not ready for their debut.

It was two days later that they had their coming out. I have to say Dr. 90210 is pretty good. There is actually something there to look at now. I just pretend there is a blurry spot over my nipples, like on TV, when they blur out someone's private parts with that fuzzy blob. You see, I don't have new nipples yet.

Which reminds me, for some reason: Go get a mammogram! That's how my cancer was found. And did I mention that they got it all? "Elvis" has left the building, if you know what I mean. Yee-Haw! Let the healing begin.

Thanks so much for everything. Thank you that I was never alone. Thank you for your prayers, support, cards, flowers, fruit, jewelry, beautiful purse, books, Christmas platter, green tea and boob key chain. Thank you for being my friend, and not just because you happen to be related.

God is good, all the time.

October 31, 2008

It's Halloween and I am already dressed in my costume. You'll know it's me if you see a trick or treat-er wearing a post-mastectomy vest under an Adidas sweat suit, bad hair, and a grimace of pain. I think there was a character much like me in "The Rocky Horror Picture Show." In fact, I think this is how I used to dress in the 1970's when we would go see that movie during the midnight showing at Woodland Theater. My poor husband probably thinks that I am having some sort of mid-life crisis, and reverting to my teenage glory days. Little does he know my hair looks like this because it just hurts so much to raise my arms above my shoulders and fix it. Oh, and I haven't taken my pain pills yet today.

Over the last week I have questioned whether or not I did the right thing having both my breasts removed. I even asked Dr. 90210's nurse what she thought when I was there earlier this week. "You did it, so it must have been the right thing to do," she said, going for tact. Ha! How trite. The verbal pathology report indicated that removing the one breast was a must, but I could have preserved the second.

I have come to a startling conclusion: I really never believed that I had cancer. I talked about it. I read about it. I shared my feelings about it. But the whole time it has been more of an out-of-body experience. Like I am talking about the Kim that is sitting next to me, not the one that currently has gas from all of the stool softeners I have been consuming.

Think about that statement: I have cancer. Who says that? Do you think that could become part of your speech, part of what you say to people? "Hello, my name is (your name here). It has been three months since my last glass of wine. I have cancer." This just does not work for me.

I was recently blessed with a wonderful new daughter-in-law to add to the two incredible ones I already had. I have grandchildren! I have a husband who cannot find anything without me. I have friends whose lives would certainly be incomplete if I wasn't there from time to time to share my view on the new fall fashions, or world peace, or whatever it is we talk about. I have a dad who has been through enough in life, and I know that I am his favorite (right?). My children seek my sage wisdom on a near-daily basis. If I am incapacitated, who would put LeeAnne's bric-a-brac in the right places? Who would laugh with Lindsey at all of the funny things that Susan says in the office? Who would my babies call "Uma"? *Who?*

I would say "I have cancer," but I never believed it. This reminds me of when I get my driver's license renewed, and I tell them my height is 5'2" and my weight is 120 pounds. The Secretary of State clerk gives me a funny look, but I stay firm. I give her the look meant to communicate *"Don't mess with me, maybe I am just a little bloated today."*

Or, what about smiling and saying "I'm fine" when you just had a big fight with your spouse, and if he knows what's good for him, he had better be on his way to pick up the kids from soccer practice bearing flowers from the store. You say it but don't believe it. Or, when you are told how great you look, and respond with "So do you," even though you know the person you are lying to looks twenty years older than she should look. We don't mean everything we say, do we?

I say "cancer," but I do not really believe it exists.

Even now I still do not believe it. I would rather say "I am going to have a fine rack when this is all said and done." Yeah, I think I will say that and it will probably be true.

In any event, God is good, all the time.

November 3, 2008

Over the last few days I have come to grips with my decision on the double removal deal. I think that when the pain subsides, and I have beautifully tattooed florescent pink nipples I will know that I did the right thing. I keep hearing stories about people that removed one, and had to go back for seconds a couple of years down the road. This way, a couple of years down the road, the pair of them will be happily tucked inside a leopard print Wonder Bra.

The pain is still there. I wish it would leave. I think it has definitely overstayed its welcome. I am horrible about taking the pills if Steve is not here. He is better than having Florence Nightingale as my nurse. He even washed my hair in the kitchen sink!

Steve makes really good oatmeal for breakfast that rivals my dad's oatmeal (and my dad is the master). He brings me my pills on time, adjusts pillows, tells me 'no' when I ask him if I smell bad, hasn't said a word about my new post-surgery hair style, washes all of the dishes, cleans the house...he does *everything*. I just hope I am the one in this marriage that becomes senile and incontinent first, because I now know what excellent care I will receive. When Steve is not around I tend to get behind on the pain meds and it can be hard to get on top of it again. I would ask him to take more time off (it's legal for a spouse to take time off work to care for a sick partner under the Family and Medical Leave Act), but since he owns the place that might not work out.

I can hardly believe that my surgery was two weeks ago. The two weeks leading up to surgery seemed like a year-and-a-half. These two weeks have been a drug induced couple of days. There are a couple of deeply personal things I have been holding onto to that I would like to now share. I wasn't sure if I would ever be at a point that I would want to, or be able to, put these things in writing. I will make an attempt, anyway.

If you have been receiving my updates for a while, you might remember that God and I had a talk back in August. As a reminder, here they are again:

"My child, listen to me. You will go through a trial, a time of mourning and sadness. But know that through it all I am by your side. At the end true happiness will be found. Do not give up, do not despair. I will be with you always. It is okay, for you have been preparing for this time. Rest in Me. Trust in Me. Stay the course. Do not waver for those around you will look to you for strength, my strength. *Let your light shine. I love you. My love is everlasting. Stay the course."*

At the time I was a bit nervous, wondering what trial I would be facing. Then I got the Big Pink Ribbon news. Even after being diagnosed, I questioned the mourning piece of God's message. I now know that I am mourning my pair of "friends" that I became extremely attached to when I found out they were taking the midnight train to Georgia.

As long as I have believed in God, I have believed that He is omnipresent. I don't know how He does it, but He is everywhere, all of the time. So, when He let me know that He would remain by my side through it all, I thought that was nice confirmation of something that I already believed. Some of what God told me, I haven't entirely figured out yet, but I am sure everything will come to light sooner or later.

Over the last couple of months, knowing that God is by my side has meant so much. When I had my first MRI (can you say "claustrophobia"?), I was praying that I would not freak out. At that moment God gently whispered in my ear that He was holding my hand. Immediately, I had peace and contentment amidst the loud banging and heat of the MRI machine. I knew then that He would hold my hand through any other procedure or surgery. What a great feeling to know that I would not being going into any of this alone, especially the surgery room, that sterile room with the bright lights and the green masked people.

There is only one thing that I remember from the recovery room after my mastectomy. I woke up shivering with my teeth clattering. A nurse placed one of those wonderful warm blankets (a wonderful invention, blanket warmers!) over me to fight the chills. I opened my eyes, and there was a man standing next to me. He was just standing there. I knew that he was not part of the medical staff because he was casually dressed, not dressed in green scrubs, and without a mask on his face.

At first I thought maybe I was seeing someone who wasn't really there. I looked away, and looked back, and there he was. Then I realized he was holding my hand. The man was not "he" but He, the Lord. Just as He promised, Jesus was there for me. I closed my eyes, and the next thing I remember Steve was by my side in the hospital room that was to become my home for the next few days.

I have thought about that moment in recovery many times over the last few weeks. When I first remembered the mysterious man, I wondered if he was just a kind man bringing me comfort, although why would he be allowed in the recovery room? I also wondered if some of the drugs that pumped through my veins had hallucinogenic properties. That doesn't totally add up either, because I know my mind was quite clear at that point. Faith tells me the man was Him, my Lord, right there with me through it all, just as He promised.

I do not know what the next step is in the whole cancer process. I am praying that when I see the oncologist on Thursday she tells me "Hey, we got it all. Nothing more needs to be done! Go in peace." I do know that I will be seeing Dr. 90210 for a while, until he lives up to his guarantee of a forever perky pair. I do know that whatever is ahead, God is by my side, just as He was in the recovery room, just as He promised.

God is good, all the time.

November 5, 2008

I am feeling pretty yucky, and it has nothing to do with the election results. The doctor told me that I could develop an infection, but that would be very rare. I am a 'rare' individual, in more ways than one. In fact, I feel so yucky that I was just wondering why my left foot was so cold. I discovered that I failed to sock up my left foot like I did my right. The sock is now on. All is well in Byron Center.

Regarding the election results, I feel proud. I am so happy to be living during a time when the shade of a person's skin does not determine his electability into the highest office in our country, and perhaps the world (second under the Pope, of course). It was not that long ago that if you were darker skinned than another, it meant you had to sit on the back of the bus, use separate toilets, eat in different eateries, be non-eligible for country club memberships etc. Quenching your thirst at the same drinking fountain as the light skinned people was strictly prohibited. I would like to believe that if I were old enough at the time, I would have marched with Dr. Martin Luther King, given up my seat on the bus, and opened my restaurant to everybody, as well as my golf course.

Praise God that the shade of a person's skin does not determine his/her value, intelligence or worthiness. And praise God that there are more of us out there who realize that. Certainly we live in a diverse world with many cultures. Part of the beauty of our country is the diversity in culture, cuisine, art, and skin shade. Who is allowed to have the arrogance to think that one style of living is better than another? I have traveled the world, and can tell you that there is something to be said for the simple life of a Peruvian Inca or Dominican farm worker. When the work day is done, it is done. No running here and there to soccer practice, dance rehearsals, the mall, the game, the bar. We think that everyone has to be on full speed, full time. Resting is alright. In fact, it is better than alright. We need to take time to reflect, talk to God, enjoy a quiet meal with someone, read a good book, rest, renew, relax, retreat, and restart. We need to relearn what life is and who people are.

God created each one of us. He loves each one of us. Just like our children are so special to us, we are so special to Him. If we could see people the way God does, I believe the world would change. There would not be so many middle fingers in rush hour traffic, or fear of people that live on our streets, judgment or condemnation.

I say good luck, Barrack Obama. Whether you voted for him or not, he is going to be our leader as of January 20th, 2009. Leaders need our prayers and support! By the way, thanks George Bush for all of the time that you put into the presidential office. I hope you enjoy retirement, and get some much deserved rest.

God is good, all the time.

November 6, 2008

Last night I visited the Emergency Room at St. Mary's Hospital. I had some pretty yellow stuff coming from places where yellow stuff shouldn't be, so the doctor thought it would be best to get things checked out. The short of it is they changed my antibiotic, and I already feel a bit better today. I will tell you the long of it some other time.

Today, I visited Dr. 90210, and was unable to expand the expanders due to the yellow stuff and lots of swelling. The funny thing is I was happy when he told me that. I still had a lot of swelling and thus a lot of pain. I was happy to know that the pain was there for good reason. Thankfully, he said this in front of Steve "Florence Nightingale" Sorrelle, which made us both think maybe I am not being such a baby after all.

I also visited Dr. "Best Ever" Caughran. She went over the pathology report with us. Apparently I had cancer in six different spots in the girl to the left. In one of the spots, the margins (the areas just beyond the cancer) weren't looking as clear as she would have liked, so she will be monitoring it for a while. The good, no, *great* news is she is 98 % "ish" sure that she got it all, so no chemo and no radiation and no Tamoxifin.

All of that add up to the following: I get to keep my hair, chest cavity, and my monthly visitor. Praise God! (I think that this is the first time I have praised God for "Aunt Flo," as they say.) Dr. Caughran also told me that I absolutely did the right thing because a mastectomy was the only way they could have gotten all of that cancer. And the whole double thing makes great sense. It's not worth it to take a chance on what is behind Curtain Number Two.

Even though right now I should be doing the dance of joy, for some reason I have this apprehension. I think it might stem from the fact that I did not even *know* that I had cancer until just a few weeks ago. The only reason I found out is because I had this mysterious elbow pain and said, "Hey Doc, since I'm here anyway, would you mind taking a look at my breasts?" The doctor examined my breasts, found a lump, and ordered me to get a mammogram. I could only feel one lump, but it was actually six growths.

How does someone have six cancerous growths, and have no idea? And what if my elbow hadn't hurt? (It was diagnosed as tennis elbow in my left elbow, which is strange because I am right handed and I have not played tennis since 2007.) Have I mentioned that God is good, all the time? I give him the credit for the early detection, due to tennis elbow, of all things!

I did the whole monthly shower routine, really I did. Check-ups, mammograms (every couple of years), read the breast cancer articles, wore the pink ribbon: I did what I thought I was supposed to do. I wish that there was a blood test, or better yet, a machine that you could walk through, like at the airport, and it has a read out: BP 120/70, temp 98.6, pulse 70, oxygen 98%, breast cancer, lose a few pounds. Wouldn't that be great? They could even have it at the airport, which could save healthcare costs, and give all those homeland security people something else to do.

I feel this way, especially since right now my mother-in-law receives the Full Monty of security checks every time we fly because of her new hip. Anyway, all I know is that I thank God that the big 'C' was discovered early enough to be contained, and taken out. Thank you Lord! I guess the lesson is to listen to that still small voice in your head. Not the one that reminds you at 11:00 p.m. that there is still some Moose Tracks Ice Cream in the freezer. I am talking about the voice that nudges you to let that elderly gentleman ahead of you in the check-out lane, call your Dad and tell him how much you love him, or go get a mammogram.

God is good, all the time.

By the way, as Maxine says "Live your life in such a way that when your feet hit the floor in the morning the devil says 'oh shoot!'" (I paraphrased the last word.)

November 11, 2008

I have been eating a lot of apples lately and believe me it is not keeping the doctors away. Yesterday, I spent some time with Dr. 90210. I am telling you, if you need your eyes lifted, lips plumped, or your breasts taken off, he is your man. I went with the intention of expanding the expanders by a couple of ounces or so but, yet again, was too swollen or whiny (I am not sure which) to get any additions. Next week I will go back and try again. I have to admit I was not looking forward to anyone putting needles in where it already hurt so much. Maybe I will be looking forward to it more next week.

I am also going to see my primary physician (I know the lingo now) on Thursday. Remember the whole elbow thing? I am going for a recheck on that, and a couple of other things. I am also visiting her because I have lost my internal thermometer. I have no idea where it went, but I am either hot or cold with no temperature in between. I used to be more like Hawaii, 80 degrees and sunny all year long. Sure, I would get cold in the winter and have to wear socks to bed, but who doesn't when you live where there are blizzards instead of tropical storms, and icicles instead of palm trees? Now I am either sweating profusely or cold enough to need not only socks, but a couple of extra blankets and a sweatshirt.

I realize that I am a woman in my forties, closing in on the Big Change. I just don't think I am old enough to be changing quite yet. I swear, it was just last week I was wearing a Comstock Park football jersey with 'Langlois' on the back of it, and cheering the Panthers on to victory. I never did wear the turtle neck with the whales on it, but you had better believe I owned Adidas T-shirts in several colors, adored the creator of platform shoes for the added inches they gave me, and had Converse All-Star high tops in my school colors.

I still wear Levi boot cut jeans, just like I did when I wasn't wearing my new designer Calvin Kleins. The only difference is, back then I would use ink to black out the size on the back tag, now I use a Sharpie.

I still own my varsity jacket in green and gold with "Kim" embroidered on the right chest, the big 'CP' underneath and a '79 on the sleeve. My medals from student council and National Honor Society are still attached. I have the playbills from my school performances as Mrs. Silvia Potter-Porter in *Annie Get Your Gun*, and will never forget Sheila hanging the star in "Coopersville" during *Bye Bye Birdie* (or was it *Carousel*? Mr. Meyers would know for sure). Okay, so the jacket doesn't fit like it used to, and the playbills are a little yellowed, but it has not been *that* long.

I have to admit that my memory seems a little affected as well. I can't recall in which play Sheila hung the star, or where I put those darn keys. I do have a theory, however. It's not memory loss, but simply brain overload. Every day of my forty seven years I have heard, watched, and learned something. Each factoid that I have gathered has been stored in the old gray matter all along. An eighteen year old only has so many files. At forty seven my drawers are just getting fuller. Until someone invents an expandable hard drive that uses an ear like a USB port, I have to call my cousin Mary to tell me who sang "We've Got Tonight," and figure out the name of Marcia Brady's date to her junior prom (Davy Jones, I think).

I am grateful that God has infinite memory. I am more grateful that His memory can be a bit selective, so that when I screw up He is quick to forgive and forget. Thanks Lord. I need to be more like you.

God is good, all the time.

P.S. It's Veteran's Day, so I just want to say thank you to all the veterans.

November 13, 2008

Today is a day for new prayer. The praying that everyone has been doing has been fantastic. It is such a great feeling to know that people are praying for me. I can feel it. My Dominican son, Cristian Santiago, wrote to tell me that he put my name on his computer so he sees it every day and remembers to pray for me. Wow--how sweet and somehow humbling to know that Cristian is praying for me so fervently.

I have also been the pray-er. People would call and say, "Hey Kim, someone needs prayer for something." I was happy to pray for every one of those requests. I passed the requests on to others, whether it was drought in Burkina Faso, malaria at the Village of Hope, my friend with cancer, someone needing work, a hurricane in the Dominican Republic...anything. I believe in prayer. God listens. And God answers. That is one of the things that I love about God, His big ears and His big heart.

I read today that God answers prayers with one of three responses:

1.   Okay.
2.   Later.
3.   I have something better in mind for you.

I have a new prayer, and new requests. I visited my Primary Care physician today, Karen Dempsey. She is the best. I am blessed with great doctors! Thank you, Lord. Anyway, I had been having some "woman issues" since before this other bump in the road happened. I had tried to push the idea of menopause out of my mind, thinking that I was years if not decades away from such a big physical change. The doctor confirmed my thoughts: I am not even close to being menopausal--yeah me!
The only problem is that the problems I am having are real problems. So, I will be going for an ultrasound soon, followed by a visit to Grand Rapids #1 OB/GYN, John LaGrand. I have known John socially for several years, besides the fact that he also delivered three of my five grandchildren and did an outstanding job. I know this because those babies are amazing.

It is just a little funny, however, to think about going to a doctor who will explore my anatomy in such a personal way, and then possibly have cake and ice cream with him at a friend's birthday party next month. I have not yet been in that position. This will be my first visit to the good doctor. Again, I have a new prayer and a new request.

I am sure that all is fine. The tiny little pit in my stomach over this has a lot to do with a few things I know. First, I am the same age as my mother was when she had her baby equipment removed because of a cyst the size of a grapefruit in her uterus.

Secondly, statistically woman in my age category who have had breast cancer are at greater risk for ovarian cancer (and colon cancer, of all things). But maybe that tiny little pit is just the last of the big pit that has been slowly leaving my stomach since my great surgery results. Plus, God is not into statistics, and He could care less that I happen to be the same age as my mom was then. He cares about me for me. He cares about my heart. I love that about God.

Depending on the ultrasound results, I will again be faced with choices. Possibly, I'll be faced with another dilemma of whether to remove or not to remove a body part or growth. Yup, I have a new prayer and a new request for you to consider.

God is good, all the time.

November 16, 2008

Weekends are great: two days of allowed laziness. I have not been going into work, so during the week I feel a little bad about that. But on the weekend I would not be going in anyway, so I am guilt free. Doctors seem to take weekends off, too. Friday test results don't come until at least Monday. No appointments, no calls. No news is good news, so I've heard. Today there is no reason to think about Friday's ultrasound results. I can wait and think about it tomorrow. *Monday*. Not the weekend.

There are two things that I really have going for me right now: my faith in God, and my friends. Last week when my daughter needed a last minute babysitter a great friend came over to help with her girls. Other assorted great friends...

• took me to lunch and the Friday ultrasound.

•brought over dinner (and dessert!) last week after looking on the internet for recipes that are friendly to my particular diet right now. I hadn't had dessert since Labor Day!

•set his computer password, so he remembers to pray for me every day.

•curled my hair. I was looking hot in my sweats and curled hair!

•watched hours of Grey's Anatomy episodes next to me in my bed, and never complained when I got too involved and started questioning Dr. McDreamy's decisions (she just blamed the pain killers).

•brought meals. Meals, for just me and Steve! Incredible. We have been eating oatmeal and salad, and our great friends have brought feasts.

•promise to continue to call every week to hear directly from me how I am feeling.

Several friends have sent me encouraging emails and cards, or pray for me "without ceasing." To wrap it up, I have really great friends, some of whom are even relatives.

I could go on and on about the wonderful things that my friends have done for me, for us. Just as I don't know how someone would get through this without faith in God, I also have no clue how someone would get through this without friends. I have friends that I have known since elementary school, and friends that I have known for just a few months. I have friends who live close by, and friends that live far away. I have friends that introduce me to other people who become my friends. I have friends that are going through hard times and friends that are on top of the world. I have old friends, new friends, green friends, blue friends.

Friends that sing.

Friends with bling.

Friends that dance.

Friends in France.

Each friend is a gift, no two with the same wrapping paper, and no repeat presents. I treasure each one. Thanks for being a friend, down the road and back again.

God is good, all the time.

November 19, 2008

I *know*. It's been two days in a row with this update business! Well, it *is* called an update, so that is what I am doing, updating.

I actually saw Dr. 91210 two days ago. The expansion began. The doctor used a magnet to find the quarter size area that they must hit so that fluid is added instead of depleted. It is pretty fascinating. There is an opening, the needle goes into the opening, they push saline through the needle and the opening closes on its own. Who comes up with this stuff? Amazing!

It is like watching a balloon expand, just a little more painful. More like watching a balloon expand while someone is running her fingernails down the chalkboard. Oh yeah, it was fun. Actually the procedure itself was pretty easy. Afterwards, however, Dr. 90210's nurses told me that I would feel some "tightness" and perhaps a little "discomfort." I was told the same thing during labor while I was strangling my husband and telling him that he could never touch me again. I had pain then, and I have pain now. Maybe I am just a baby, but I did take pills. And I did whine a bit to Steve. Steve listened. He is good at that. He couldn't really do anything for me, but I have to say that when he told me a hot bath was waiting, I almost ran to get there. Those of you who live in real winter weather know how great a hot bath feels after a cold day. It is better than Vicodin and Valium together.

Next Tuesday I go for a refill. This week the doctor put in about 50cc's on each side. Next week they will be putting 100 cc's on each side. Steve, you had better have that bath ready. Please, baby? Bubbles would be nice this time.

I told Dr. 90210 that I call him Dr. 90210. He already knew, as he had talked to a friend of mine, Ann, who told him of the reference. He thought it was because he has sideburns. I told him that it has nothing to do with his sideburns. I am now under the assumption that plastic surgeons do not have time for TV, at least not reality television. He probably watches shows like "Grey's Anatomy" and "House" to learn new diagnostic and surgical skills. I also told him that my Primary Care Physician said that I looked the best, reconstructive-wise, she had ever seen anyone look who had had surgery so recently.

Dr. 90210 is humble, but I think he knows how good he is. He's not like Dr. Rey; he is more like that really nice doctor that has a wife and a baby on the show "Dr. 90210." Humble and great are two virtues nice to have in a doctor. Next Monday afternoon I will be seeing Dr. John LaGrand, GYN Surgeon. I was asked what kind of a nickname he will have. I already know him and know that he is good. So Dr. "Not-So-Grand" would be completely inappropriate. I will give it some thought.

I read something today that summed up, for me, life's bottom line. In the words of Rick Warren, "We were made by God and for God, and until you figure that out, life isn't going to make sense. Life is a series of problems: you are in one now, you're just coming out of one, or you're getting ready to go into another one. The reason for this is that God is more interested in your character than your comfort. God is more interested in making your life holy than He is in making your life happy. We can be reasonably happy here on earth, but that's not the goal of life. The goal is to grow in character, in Christ likeness."

I believe God looks at not what we do, but how we do it. He doesn't look at how many hungry kids we feed, but rather looks at our heart to feed them. He doesn't pay attention to the words we say to our friends, but how we say them. He looks at our response to the crap more than he looks at the crap. He's not as concerned with how we fill our day as he is with our gratitude for another day. I believe that when we know we are not just created by God, but *for* Him, then naturally we will love our creator. Love is a vow, not just an emotion. When you say you love someone you are committing to treat them right, hold them up in hard times, celebrate with them during good times, for better or worse, richer or poorer. Love is a vow.

Loving God is a vow, one of submission to His will and to being a reflection of His love. I love God. I take that vow.

God is good, all the time.

November 21, 2008

It is amazing how many names I have acquired in my life. At birth I was given the name Kimberly Sue Langlois, Kimmie for short. My aunts, uncles and cousins still call me Kimmie. Starting in kindergarten, I became Kim to the non-family world. When I would have a spat with the neighbor kids, I became "Lead Bottom Langlois," to which I would respond "Cigar Butt Garstka!" Once, while playing kickball, I was told that my friend's mother wears army boots (I never saw Mrs. Eister in army boots. Maybe she just wore them when family was around).

I will never forget being called "pleasantly plump" as an eight-year-old. At Holy Trinity Middle School, I was a "Condor," and at Comstock Park High School, I became a "Panther" when playing or watching sports. Other names have popped up over the years:

"Hey Waitress!"

"Mrs. Sorrelle"

"Coach"

"Mother-in-law"

"Head Chef and Bottle Washer"

Two of my favorite names are "Wife" and "Mom." Recently, I acquired a new name: "Uma." That is what my grandbabies call me (except for Evayah who calls me "Frampa," but she isn't even two yet).

I think I like "Uma" best. The name makes me feel like I have accomplished something. My kids have grown-up, moved, married, and reproduced. They have jobs and bills and couches and washing machines and spatulas. Who would have thought when their worlds revolved around Donkey Kong, Big Wheels, and T-Ball, that someday they would become heads of families with spatulas?

I wear "Uma" like a badge of honor. I love hearing Aurora say, "Uma, I love you so much," or when Crichton says, "When you coming my house, Uma?" Hearing "Uma" makes me do crazy things like color princesses, make play-dough caterpillars, watch *The Wiggles*, and have crumbs in my bed. I have no control over giving them candy, letting them watch cartoons, or when they should go to bed. Somehow, I am not able to say "no" when a question starts with "Uma, can I...?"

I now need "Uma" fixes. It is like a drug that changes my voice, vocabulary, and judgment. I no longer believe in spankings or sending kids to their rooms. Time-outs are shorter than they should be, but I know that I got my point across. After all, I hear "sorry, Uma," and all is forgiven. "Uma" turns me into a blob of flesh with a permanent smile. I love being Uma.

On October 21, 2008, I was given a new name: "Breast Cancer Survivor." This new name is music to my ears. A dear friend gave me a picture that says, "You are an inspiration to those who know you, walking in faith, seeking God's strength." This brings me to the very best and highest name I have, "Christian." I pray that I wear "Christian" on my sleeve, my shoes, my hands, my heart, and my head. I pray for God's eyes so that I can see people the way He does. I pray for God's heart, so I can have compassion, love and respect for everyone. I pray that people can see God in me. I pray that everyone can recognize how much God loves them. I pray that I am not a hindrance, but a help to God. I pray that God takes the worst of situations and makes great things come from them. I pray for healing, peace, joy, and understanding. (I kind of skip praying for patience. I learned from my Dad, you get what you ask for.)

"For I know the plans I have for you, says the Lord" (Jeremiah 29:11). Praise God! The verse goes on to say, "They are plans for good and not for evil, to give you a future and a hope."

God is good, all the time.

November 24, 2008

Today I met with Dr. John LaGrand, OB/GYN surgeon. I had a hard time finding something to wear. Jeans do not fit the same 30 pounds lighter. If boobs were a state of the union, I started with Alaska and ended up with Rhode Island. Not only are they smaller but they are lumpy. I chose some "fat" pants (that is how we overweight people refer to our clothes that we are now too small for, and hope never fit us again, but are afraid to throw away, just in case), and a sweater that hangs to my knees. I look like a little girl trying on clothes in her grandma's closet. My hair is clean, dry and curled, a feat I have accomplished alone for only the second time post-surgery. I even wore a little make-up. You are welcome, Doctor!

I finally came up with a nickname: Dr. McAnalogy (Dr. LaGrand, aka Dr. McAnalogy, because he is the king of them.) I have never known anyone who can come up with spur-of-the-moment analogies like John, except maybe Tom Maas, also a king but not a doctor. Plus, I am married, old enough to be his mother, I see him socially sometimes and probably am his oldest patient, so calling him another McDreamy, though maybe appropriate, is really very inappropriate.

He told me that with the kind of breast cancer I had, my ovaries are a ticking time bomb (his words). Dr. McAnalogy compared it to running back and forth at a shooting range: you are bound to get hit sometime. (I told you, he's the king of analogies.) My cancer was estrogen-driven, ovaries make estrogen, thus, take those suckers out and don't worry about future estrogen-driven cancers. So, I had breast cancer because of my ovaries. Or is it because I have ovaries I had breast cancer? Whichever, the end result is the same. It starts with a couple of small cuts and ends with hot flashes.

My surgery (oh, joy) will probably be on January 9, 2009. Dr. McAnalogy said that the surgery is not an emergency, but there is "urgency." Right now his office is trying to coordinate the surgery with a surgeon who will do a colonoscopy at the same time (got to love that too!), a Dr. VanderKlok or something like that. Imagine, a West Michigan doctor with "Vander" at the beginning of his name--amazing. The good news is that I get a two-for-one use of general anesthesia. By the way, did you know that the stuff you have to drink the day before a colonoscopy is called *Flagyl*? I have to say there is nothing appetizing about anything named Flagyl. Let the good times roll.

Cancer has changed me. I am concerned about certain things that never used to bother me before, while things that used to bother me no longer do. Dishes in the sink really bother me, but there are days my primping consists of little more than combing my hair. Things out of place drive me crazy, but I would be fine with living in a sweat suit for the rest of my life. Right now, getting 'dressed up for company' means wearing sweats that match. There is something about disorder that is not my friend right now. I can live with mess if I am the one creating it, but then it needs to be taken care of when I am done. Interestingly, I handled disorder better before the big "C" came into my life.

I believe I am starting to drive my immediate family crazy. My daughter came over with the babies and I ran behind them putting things back where they belonged. I told my youngest son that it's great that he comes home for weekends, but he has to put everything away that he touches. He might not even be the one touching it, but I need to have it put away. My husband knows about this new obsession, and is great about putting things back where they belong (if I don't count his dirty socks and unmentionables on the bathroom floor).

I think it is a control issue. There are things in my life that I have no control over: babies spilling a little apple juice onto the floor, how my grandson says fire truck with two f's and no t or r, my recently overactive tear ducts, and needing another surgery. So, the things that I can control, I *need* to control.

Control. I have been taught that that is something that you give up when you surrender your life to the Lord. I think that's not quite right. Control remains in our hands, but we just rethink how we are going to use it. I still have a will of my own but I want to know if it runs parallel to God's will. I still have to put one foot in front of the other, but I want to know if God is on the same path. I believe there are things that people have to give up control over to go on living, such as a grown child's decisions, past mistakes, other people's past mistakes. In general, control stays with me, the Control Giver is just who I am now aiming to please.

God is good, all the time.

November 25, 2008

Expansion number two took place this morning, courtesy of Dr. 90210. His nurse told me that he wanted to be called Dr. 49503. I am thinking about it. I am in pain. Thinking and pain do not play good together. They are both so selfish. Pain tries to control every part of you. Pain can be in a tooth yet impair your driving. Thinking does not like interruption. Thinking likes to be alone and requires quiet. Pain is loud.

It seems that Grand Rapids has quite the web of MDs. Dr. 90210 is buddies with Dr. McAnalogy. Dr. McAnalogy works with his wife, also a doctor. Dr. Mrs. Dr. McAnalogy is friends with the greatest oncology surgeon, Dr. Caughran (pronounced 'car in' as in "I put my 'car in' the garage"). I got Dr. Caughran's name from my sister-in-law, Andi, who happens to be really good friends with Dr. Mrs. Dr. McAnalogy. Dr. Caughran is in the same building with Dr. 90210. I think somehow now I am either their cousin or a doctor, too.

I got the confirmation call from Dr. McAnalogy's office that surgery will be on January 9, 2009. The hardest part of planning, apparently, was coordinating with a colonoscopist (is that the right word? I won't tell you what my sister-in-law calls such doctors, but it starts with 'a' and ends with a couple of s's.) I will let you know if I decide to have an ovary going away party. I might not, with the holiday busyness and all. Plus the only ones who will notice that I no longer have ovaries and a uterus will be the people that hear me growl. Not quite the same as losing what I used to wrap in Victoria's Secret lace.

I will begin to do research on the effects of being thrown into menopause. The word broken down is:

"Men," as in the lucky gender that does not have to go through menopause.

"O" for *"Oh no, what the heck is happening to her?"*

"Pause," as in *"stop, and run the other way because your body will never be the same again"*.

The benefits are obvious: I can sell my stock in Playtex and Midol. The list of negatives are, unfortunately, also obvious: sweating, moodiness, difficulty losing weight (as if it could get any harder!), losing all ability to bear children (maybe that is a benefit?), hair loss, and several more yet to be revealed to me. I do wonder if being thrown in is different than going in gradually and gracefully. Yesterday Dr. McAnalogy said, "You have two choices. You can have them removed and be launched into menopause and live, or you can keep them, go into menopause naturally, and take a big chance that you will die." So delicately put. I chose option number one, so, launched I will be. I am thankful for hair dye and Botox, two organic wonders that can do wonders for a lady.

My pain pills are starting to hit me hard. It is time to drift off into La La Land. I thank God for pain medicine a lot. Thanks Lord, you're the best.

God is good, all the time.

November 27, 2008

Happy Thanksgiving! When I was young this was also the day that began Christmas season. Now, green and red decorations are in stores well before Halloween, and Santa even makes it to some 4th of July parades. Like the song says, "It's the hap-happiest time of the year." I love the decorations, snow, eggnog and chestnuts roasting on an open fire. I look forward to seeing relatives that slow down for one day to catch up on family news from the whole year. Going to the mailbox is exciting, opening cards from people I love. Shopping online has made Christmas shopping extra fun. I can buy toys, pajamas, lobster, cars and power tools without leaving the comfort of my home. And then everything is delivered by those wonderful elves in brown, the UPS guys, right to my front door. Susie does the entire gift wrapping (thank you Lord for sending Susie to Noah and not just for the gift wrapping). Everyone pitches in with decorations. There are cookies to bake, people to see, places to go, things to do, Christmas TV specials to watch, trees to trim, and tears to shed.

Tears. Everyone seems to have some holiday tears, usually because someone they love has passed on or moved on, and that loss is so much harder at Christmas. I have tears even today, the day set aside to give thanks. And I do give thanks for countless things, such as family, friends, a home, food, surviving 2008, wonderful women in my life, the love of a father and the love of a Father. Truly, I am blessed far beyond whatever blessings it is I would have imagined. Thank you everyone and thank you Lord.

My tears are from loss. I lost my mom in 1990 when I was just twenty nine-years-old. My mom was great. She was very athletic so she would play driveway basketball with us, and hit baseballs in the street until one of us reached 500. When she coached basketball at Holy Trinity, I went to every practice and every game before I was even old enough to play. When it finally was my turn to play, she stepped down to a younger team so it wouldn't look like I was being favored. She recruited the best coach she knew to take her place, my Uncle Chuck. Her coaching even followed me into high school, until it became too hard to coach a team and be able to see me play at the same time. She gave up coaching, which she loved, just to make sure that she would never miss one of my games. She came to every basketball game, volleyball game, and softball game as well as every play, musical, awards banquet and school ceremony that I was ever involved in. She did the same for my brothers. Bruce golfed and played tennis, typically not high school spectator sports, but my mom went when she could anyway. She was there when Joel was taken off the football field on a stretcher heading for the hospital in a neck brace. She was there when Bruce sang "There's No Business like Show Business" in "Annie Get Your Gun." She watched Joel run track and play baseball. She would make me a bed on the couch if I had to stay home sick from school. Then she would make me milk toast and watch "Password" with me.

She did laundry and made tuna casserole, Chef Boyardee Spaghetti, and Hamburger Helper. During Lent she tried to get creative with creamed tuna on toast and pancakes for dinner. I was always allowed to have friends over, even to spend the night. My friends called her "Mom" because they were as close to her as I was. That is what she knew about being a mom: being there for me and my brothers and our friends. Whether it was driving over to my house because I had to rush one of my kids to the hospital, playing cards all Sunday afternoon while the men watched football (and snored), or helping me pack to move to a new place, she was always there for me. That was her way. That is what she knew. Maybe she wasn't a hugger, and perhaps her patience could run a bit thin, but I can still hear her laugh. Her laugh would light up a room. I still see her smile. It's her great smile I miss the most. She knew how to plan a party and get the extended family together. She was the glue.

Things kind of went bad for her after Hurricane Hugo hit while she was in St. Croix on vacation. After her hysterectomy, her doctor didn't follow up the way he should with hormone replacement for her. And then there was her drinking. In the end, I think her downfall was a combination of those three things, but the drinking was the worst of it. In a crowd, she could drink and be happy. Alone, she would drink and be miserable.

That night she was miserable. That night she was alone, as she chose to be alone. By then she was pushing everyone away, even me, her only daughter, the one who possibly could have helped her. That is the way she chose to leave us, alone and lonely for her.

The next morning after that night, my dad found her in her garage. Joel called to tell me the news, not wanting to do it over the phone but knowing he couldn't wait. My neighbors graciously watched my children as I drove in shock to my parents' house. To this day I have no idea what her note said, the one that was addressed to my dad and left on his kitchen counter. It is still the worst day of my life. I got there and my dad was a mess. He couldn't even stand up for more than a minute. I sat down and prayed with him. I begged the Lord to give us a sign that she didn't really mean to do it. I needed to know that she would not leave me that way. She was a grandmother, a wonderful grandmother, why would she do that to my kids?

Just then Bruce walked in and asked about the car keys. Steve and Joel were there too and none of them knew anything about the keys. Steve said that the car was not running when he arrived. Bruce went back into the garage and found the keys in her hands. She didn't mean to do it. See, that is what happens with carbon monoxide, you get tired and fall asleep. She was just going to sleep for a while and then go in and tear up the note. But she didn't wake up. She just slept in that white Mustang with the red convertible top. It must have been a comfortable seat. It was her last seat here, with us, on earth.

I miss her so much.

At 29, I had just begun to recognize her wisdom. I had just begun to appreciate her for who she was instead of who she wasn't. I was beginning to learn more about her childhood, something she didn't talk about much. The insights into the girl who was my mom showed me so much about the woman who was my mom. But, no matter who she was or wasn't, she was there, always, for everything, good or bad, victory or defeat, pain or joy. She was there. I miss her dearly.

During the holidays I miss her the most. She wasn't much of a baker, but she made a mean batch of eggnog and always participated in the season with great holiday cheer. As Santa, and later just as mom, she spoiled my brothers and me like crazy. She kept the tradition going by spoiling her grandchildren. I hope to follow in her footsteps. She was the party girl. She was the glue.

I am not the only one that misses her; and she is not the only one I miss. Everyone misses someone. She is just the one I miss the most. Here's to you Mom. Happy Thanksgiving. Jesus, please give my mom a big hug for me. Love you both.

God is good, all the time.

December 1, 2008

My next surgery is not until January 9, but I spent part of this weekend practicing for menopause. I saw a card with the "Seven Dwarfs of Menopause" pictured on the cover. I don't remember their names exactly, but they were something like Itchy, Bitchy, Forgetful, Grumpy, Flashy, Weepy and Pudgy.
I believe that Forgetful has a twin named You Never Told Me That. Not only do I forget, but many times I don't even

remember what it is that I am forgetting. Weepy came to visit on Thanksgiving, thus the two hours of tears that I shed writing such an uplifting update last Thursday. Bitchy is an easy one for me; now I just get to blame it on something physical. Pudgy better keep his ugly face far, far away. I did not partake in the stuffing, pumpkin pie, mashed potatoes, or any of the really good stuff that makes Thanksgiving a glutton's paradise. Hopefully all of the dwarfs have now gone back to their little house in the woods, and will leave me alone for a while.

Today might be my last expansion day. Oh boy! Right now my chest is very oddly shaped. I need to ask Dr. 90210-49503 why so much of my breasts seem to linger under my arm pits. I think these new breasts cover more chest area than the old ones, and so far do not go forward as much. Not that I want them to go forward a lot; I do want to see my toes. But forward seems natural, and natural is good.

My granddaughter, Aurora, knows that Uma has "owie boobies." She has been very gentle, but she is extremely curious. She wants to see them often, as much as I allow. Every time I show her my reconstructed girls, she says, "Uma, there's no red on it." She is only three years old, and already knows that they are missing something in the center. I will have to stick with reddish color tattoos after they are inked, because glow-in-the-dark, florescent green nipples might really freak her out.

I have heard, by the way, that once I get the new chest installed, I will never have to wear a bra. They just stay right there, in place, constantly at attention for my whole life. I will be the perkiest ninety-year-old woman on the block. While everyone else is tucking their boobs into their elastic waist bands, mine will be at full mast, proud to be American, saluting our soldiers, and anyone else who happens by. No more bra straps digging into my shoulders, no more bra lines in the back of my shirts. Not a bad perk, I'd say.

I'll take what I can get. This perk might be almost better than pumpkin pie. By the way, I hope there is pumpkin pie in Heaven. And not just pumpkin pie, but all of the foods that are no longer a part of my cancer diet. I enjoy eating. The tags on the back of my pants will tell you that. God knows a lot of us, if not all of us, enjoy a good meal. Hopefully, Heaven features eating. I would love to sit down with you there and enjoy some great food and some great conversation. Somehow here, time goes by so quickly that there are not enough of those laid back meals to enjoy.

It would be great if the meal we have together in Heaven could be at a quiet table not waiting for the next guest to be seated. There's nothing worse than growing hoarse talking over all of the background noise as the waiter keeps giving you meaningful looks to keep it moving. I want to make a reservation in a quiet spot with angels singing in the background and no one pushing us out. The best part would be in knowing we are in a place surrounded by people we love, and people we have yet to meet, celebrating together in peace and harmony forever. Let me know when you are free for dinner.

God is good, all the time.

December 2, 2008

Happy Day After Expansion Day! I came home from the doctor and took two pain killers. The pain did not go away, but the pills made me not care about it as much. Sleep is difficult with pain. It is not so much about the sleep as it is trying to get comfortable in bed. Extra pillows help. Okay, I am done whining now.

I asked Dr. 90210-49503 why the ladies go side to side more than forward. It seems that expanders do not respond to gravity like the natural ones do. Apparently the permanent ones act more like the real deal. Have I mentioned that they now come in "Round" or—new!—"Teardrop"? Another decision, but this one will be easy. I will be going with the "Teardrop." I think, maybe, unless the "Round" would be better.

This morning my dad came over for breakfast. We had a good cry over what I wrote about my mom in my Thanksgiving entry. He pointed out to me that he was the one who found my mom. For eighteen years he has been living with "What if?" I have too, and probably my brothers deal with this also. Eighteen years is a long time to kick one's self. After a while both your foot and your bottom get awfully sore. Yet the kicking continues. But I believe it has to stop.

Today is the day. Today, for the umpteenth time, I will lay it all at the foot of God and ask Him to carry the "what if?" burden for me. God will say "yes" without hesitation. Then we will have a little tug-of-war while I decide that regarding my mom's choice, there were too many outside factors I had no control over, and it wasn't my fault.

Then I will let go and let God. I hope that my Dad and my brothers do the same. But this time I want it to be different. I want to put it there and leave it there. It really wasn't anyone's fault. Not my dad's, not mine, not my brothers'. My mom made a decision that we all have to live with, including her, in Heaven.

Why is it that we need to place blame when something happens? Someone beats their wife, and it is his father's fault because he watched his dad do the same to his mom. Americans gain weight and it is McDonalds fault for Super-sizing their meals. Smokers blame Big Tobacco's appeal to youth. Hot coffee spills and burns because the fast food chain made it too hot. I would get upset about something, and my husband would blame PMS (alright, that one might be true). My point is blame is the game we play. Don't things ever just happen?

Do we not have to take responsibility for ourselves—ever? Maybe someone just slipped because they lost their balance, and it really wasn't some invisible thing in the aisle at Wal-Mart. Perhaps the wife beater and pedophile can decide to break the chain of destruction instead of reenacting it. Sometimes it is better to say 'no' to super-sizing.

Stuff happens. It just does. Blaming leads to bitterness. Bitterness leads to grumpy old people. Grumpy old people make everyone miserable. Then the people they are making miserable blame the grumpy old people for their misery. Round and round it goes. Let's throw a wrench in it. Let's stop the blame wheel, and deal with stuff when it happens instead of trying to figure out who to blame.

I know that some people blame God for things like cancer. Maybe some people need to be angry at someone and God is an easy target. So far I have not targeted God. I understand the blame, but I don't understand it at the same time. God is there, for us. Created us, loves us. I think when I cry, God cries with me. When I am in pain, He understands because He knows pain. After all, He was born in a stable, not a birthing room at Spectrum Hospital.

Shortly after He was born His family had to move for fear of His death, before He was even out of diapers. He grew up in a very hard time, a time of religious persecution, a time when

Herod told everyone that he was god and must be obeyed, a time of slavery, poverty, and pain. Then, at the young age of thirty three, He was beaten within an inch of His life, nailed to a cross to suffer not only physical agony, but public humiliation. To top it all off they put a spear into His side.

God knows pain. God knows suffering, humiliation, condemnation, blame, false accusations, and hunger. God knows it all because He lived it all. Just because He understands it does not mean He likes it or creates it. But He *gets* me when I cry. He knows my pain. He understands how important it is to laugh. He sets the bar high when it comes to love. He loves me. I love Him. He gets me.

God is good, all the time.

December 4, 2008

This time I did not cry.

It was a while ago. I won't tell you exactly when because I want to be a bit more sensitive to my husband's privacy. I wondered if I would cry. Before when I did I never saw it coming. I was so afraid that it would hit me out of the blue like the last time. The tears never came. We talked and laughed and just held on to each other for a long time after. It was great, comforting, loving, and hopeful. At that time we knew that Doctor Number One was fairly confident that she had removed all of the cancer. We did not yet know about the whole ovary thing. So we were blissful—painful, but blissful.

Sometimes I feel like I am living in limbo. I want to move on with life but feel stifled by all of this medical stuff. I want to make plans. I want to go back to work. I want to find an X-ray machine, and send a container full of medical supplies to Pastor Michel & Lydia in Ouagadougou. I want to go see all of the wonderful things that Cristian has accomplished in the Dominican Republic. I want to go back to New Orleans and help with more Katrina clean up. I want to clean closets at home. I want to see my son & daughter-in-law's apartment in Kalamazoo. I want to go to Hawaii. I want to go to Burkina Faso with my uncle. Maybe all of those things are not wants but needs. I need to do those things. I need to be used. But instead I am in this prison that is my body. I am trying to do all I can to regain energy and strength, but then it will start all over with the next surgery, then the next. The plans that I make lately have to do with which doctor's office on what day of the week followed by what medication.

Freedom is not what it used to be. I live in America, own a car, can afford gas, come and go as I please. Not anymore. My freedom now is limited to the walls of my house, the whims of my drivers, and the way I feel.

I had decided not to put up Christmas decorations, but am now regretting that decision. I may not do the tree but I am going to get out some of the other frou-frou as my energy allows. When you have had the 'C' word in your life, it is not difficult to guilt someone into helping bring boxes up from the basement. (I would have made a great Jewish mother! Actually, I think I am a Jewish mother. We have the same God.) The most aggressive decision that I have made in the past few months is to put off my ovarian abduction until after Christmas. I did not want to cancel our family trip to New York. Eight days with no doctors! No offense Docs, but I could use a break.

I am sure that others going through something like this feel the same. One day at a time. In the wisdom of the big Book we are told not to look to tomorrow because tomorrow has enough trouble of its own. Isn't that the truth?

Holy cow! If we knew all the trouble we were in for down the road, we would probably never leave the house. And the past, well, it is in the past. I remember years ago hearing Mark Lowry say that his favorite verse in the Bible is "it came to pass." Everything comes to pass. The highest of highs and the lowest of lows are here, then gone. Just like you cannot dance at your son's wedding forever, you also cannot grieve at your mother's grave forever.

Life moves on. Praise God. Wallowing is tough and celebrating is tiring. The in-between times are pretty good. The in-between times are for refreshing, renewing, resting, retreating, restarting. The only problem with the in-between is knowing there is another mountain or a valley around the corner.

I praise God for the valleys that make me stronger, the mountains that make me fuller and the in-between times that make me renew.

God is good, all the time.

December 6, 2008

Why is it that my grandbabies are cutest when they are sleeping? Maybe it is because I am on Day Four of babysitting for my daughter. She has two children: Aurora (named after Sleeping Beauty), three, and Cordelia (one of King Lear's daughters, and also a moon around Uranus. Hopefully she is named after the princess), twenty months. I cannot yet lift either one of them without pain. I cannot yet hug them the way an

Uma is supposed to, smothering them in between two large lumps of love. Aurora understands but little Cordelia has no idea.

With only 18 more shopping days until Christmas, people are worrying about what gift to buy whom, when cookies will be baked, and the extra price of postage for cards. All that concerns Aurora is what Sponge Bob will be doing today. Oh, the innocence of youth! No wonder Jesus said "Let the little children come to me."

I'd rather have the joy of children nearby than the endless issues of adulthood. The biggest decision Aurora has to make is whether she will have apple juice or milk with her lunch. Money issues, family issues, job issues make people go nuts. Then something hits, out of the blue, like the way that football hit "The Brady's Bunch's" Marcia in the nose. That's when you learn to appreciate youth and life and what life is really all about.

Aurora was there on September 5, which was Diagnosis Day. I was babysitting. Aurora and Cordie were in the bathtub. I knew I would be getting the biopsy results and had a big knot in my stomach, not just a simple square knot but one of those fancy knots that only sailors and magicians know how to make. My son, Noah, was helping with the girls. The phone rang. I cried at the news. For a moment I forgot that the babies were in the bathtub.

The other day Aurora said, "Uma doesn't cry anymore." At first, I didn't know what she was talking about. Then it hit me, like Marcia's football.

Emotions are crazy things. I cry every year when I watch "It's a Wonderful Life." And I laugh out loud when I watch The Office. Every year on my mom's birthday I get cranky and don't realize the date until the next day. I can't begin to explain holiday emotions.

Since September 5, I laugh harder, even at things that used to make my eyes roll. I now recognize the beauty of snow falling, Christmas lights twinkling and the babies sleeping. Juicy red grapefruit and sugar free Jell-O put a smile on my face. Talking with a friend has greater value. Since September 5, I hardly notice Steve's snoring or what size pants I am wearing. I guess sometimes it takes a football to the head to realize how great life really is.

God is good, all the time.

My Christmas Prayer
December 8, 2008

Alright Lord, I know what I want for Christmas: a miracle.

I have been watching a few Christmas movies on Hallmark and Lifetime and see miracles happen like crazy. The choir of homeless men is granted a rare license to sing in the New York subway, an angel is sent down to a man who wishes he'd never been born, the unlikely meeting of what becomes the perfect couple, an angry old woman finds purpose and joy again in the friendship of an eight-year-old-girl. The list of Christmas miracles goes on and on.

I have a few miracle requests of my own. My friend, Karen, has a brain tumor. I would like that to be taken away, please. Karen is fighting, but everyone gets tired of fighting.

I have a friend who has a beautiful 13-year-old daughter, Hannah, who has cancer. They are all fighting for Hannah. They are trying everything they can to help her. I want her cancer packaged up and thrown into a raging inferno, never to hurt her or anyone else again. My husband's cousin, Dave, is going through chemo right now for colon cancer. I want to see his body healed and all of the cancer taken away.

Three gifts, three miracles — that's not too much to ask, is it?

You saw the truckload of gifts I received every year as a child, so you realize, for me, three is a pretty small number. But that's really all that I want. Oh, and Lord, you do not have to wait until Christmas Day. Life gets so busy around the holidays, with family parties, shopping, cooking, baking, decorating, celebrating, rejoicing, singing, praising, watching cheesy movies on T.V. Darn! There is hardly time for cleaning the toilets. So anytime between now and the celebration of Your Son's birth would be great.

I have seen your miracles, firsthand. I have witnessed your love and your power. I believe that with a touch, a word, a smile, miracles happen. Miracles happen every day. Sometimes we see them: a woman with MS dancing down the aisles of church, an X-ray showing no signs of cancer, seizures stopping, a baby, born with cancer and not expected to live, has grown up and will soon be celebrating his twentieth Christmas.

Sometimes we do not see the miracles, but they happen anyway. Miracles happen, in a wounded man finding love again in a wounded woman, the car accident avoided because your phone rang just as you were walking out the door, the twenty dollar bill found on the street by the single mom wondering where dinner was going to come from that night.

Miracles are precious to me. Please Lord, give us the faith of a child, a faith that is not cynical, does not depend on logic and reasoning, a faith that is just pure and deep and trusting. Give us your peace that surpasses all understanding in a time of unrest and discontent. Please give us wisdom, your wisdom, as we make decisions for ourselves and others. Lord, pour out your unconditional love that helps us better love others. Thank you for your forgiveness. Help us to forgive as you do. Father, please touch Karen, Hannah and Dave. Bring them healing. Bring them a Christmas miracle. Thank you.

God is good, all the time.

December 10, 2008

Something very shocking happened yesterday. While I was chatting with Dr. 90210-49503 during what was finally, really my last expansion, I asked him a question to which I was sure I already knew the answer. I asked the good doctor if he was finished with his Christmas shopping and he should have replied, "Are you kidding me? I run to Meijer just before they close on Christmas Eve." (Actually, being a plastic surgeon maybe he would run to DeVries Jewelers or at least hit the jewelry counter at Meijer rather than the small home appliance department.)

Instead, while injecting saline into my right breast, he said, "Oh yeah, I've been done for a while. I love to buy gifts." What? Not only is he causing me physical pain but he made my head hurt. I did not know that any man shopped before December 24. I do not know these men. I do not live with these men. I am not related to these men in any way. I wonder if they all look the same. Maybe. I also wonder if they do dishes. Hmmm...

Because yesterday was my last fill-up, I will not be seeing a doctor until December 29. On that day I will find out when the new tear shaped models will be installed. Dr. 90210-49503 told me that they look and feel pretty real which I interpret as pretty spectacular. I still have not decided on a tattoo color, but I have picked a size.

I have heard that there are several emotional stages that a person experiences when faced with a tough diagnosis. I have read the experts list of stages, but I have my own. I realize that I am not a medically trained person, but with my real life experience, I believe my list is pretty darn accurate. Stages one through six:

- Shock
- Sadness
- Disbelief
- Frustration
- Grief
- Anger

These six stages occur between the day you are diagnosed and continue until the end of day three. Stage seven is heavy medical investigation brain overload. The eighth stage rears its ugly head somewhere in the middle of stage seven: mourning your two breasts. Nine, dancing like a crazy woman, and then praying like a sane one, happens just before surgery. Stage ten is pain, which comes after they wake you up with your new breasts. Right now, I have one foot in stage ten and the other in stage eleven, which is grumpiness. Let's just call it "Grumpy."

Pain makes me grumpy. I am not great at grumpy. In fact, there may be people around me that might mistake Stage Grumpy as unkind, short tempered or even on the edge of bitchy. Hard to believe, but I am afraid it is true. I will be happy when stages ten and eleven are over, as will everyone with whom I come in contact. I will keep you posted so that you know when to approach me. If anyone has an extra bed for

Steve, I am sure that he would be most grateful. As time goes on, I am sure that the rest of the stages will be revealed to me. Right now, I am taking pills to kill stage ten and trying hard to step on the head of stage eleven.

As I write this, it is the first time I have been alone in eight days. I have babysat two granddaughters for eight days in a row. Not all day, not without help (thank you!) but every day, for eight days, more than a week straight, there have been babies here, every day. They are good babies. They are cute babies. But they are babies. Diapers, naps, meals, baths, runny noses, cartoons, toys, stuffed animals, for eight days. My vocabulary suffered, my sleep suffered, my mind suffered, and then those around me suffered. I blamed the meds, but really it was the babies.

I am alone, but not really. I have seen a couple of those movies where the moronic high school girl walks into a dark, vacant house alone where the madman in the mask is lying in wait. I don't like that kind of alone. I do like the alone that I feel when I am physically alone but know that God is here, with me. When I pray He hears me. When I ask, He answers me. When I cry, He holds me. When I laugh, He smiles.

God is good, all the time.

December 15, 2008

Do you ever receive those emails that you must read, pass on to six people, spin around four times, eat a grapefruit, and within twenty four hours something great will happen in your life? I never pass those on but somehow I have hit the jackpot anyway! My son, Luke, is in the nuclear program in the U.S. Navy. He is second in his class, and why wouldn't he be, with bright parents, good schooling (thank you Tri-Unity), and a great work ethic?

Even though he was not supposed to receive any time off for Christmas, we are flying to New York today to see him briefly and spend a week with the rest of our kids, spouses, grandkids and G.G. (Steve's mom goes by G.G., which stands for Great Grandma). The jackpot happened yesterday when Luke was informed by the powers that be that he would have ten days off starting on December 18 and concluding on December 29! Now, the whole family will be there, together, for the better part of a week. Did I tell you that God is good, all the time?

Our plane leaves at noon today. G.G. will get the full pat down in security due to her new hip. She really doesn't seem to mind it. I always watch just to see if the security agent is going to get to second base.

I am wondering if I will get a "cheap date" today as well. There are metal pieces imbedded in my chest now, pieces that Dr. 09210 uses to locate the opening of my expanders, one on each side. If the metal beeps and the security people tell me, "Step aside, miss," I will somehow need to explain metal in my chest. Certainly people have flown with such things before, right? I don't think that I fit the description of a terrorist, whatever that is anymore. But since I am not in possession of card, like G.G. has, with a picture of her new hip, and I can't blame the beeps of the wand on an underwire bra, I can't predict how the experience will pan out.

I am hoping that leaving Michigan and getting some distance between myself and doctors will make the pain go away. I am looking forward to being with everyone, playing cards and Scrabble, reading books and relaxing. I will be doing all of those things under the influence of a little white pill if the pain is still there. But that is alright, because I laugh a bit more on the white pill. I think I am funnier and deeper, though sometimes I notice that those around me do not necessarily understand the depths of my humor—their laughter can be rather subdued.

Someday they will suddenly understand the jokes and laugh out loud. I think. Or maybe someday I will understand that I really wasn't terribly funny after all, and appreciate their kind, pity chuckles. Either way, I will have a great time.

Steve and I attended First Assembly yesterday. Pastor Sam talked about the lineage of Jesus. There were some incredible men in Jesus' lineage, and also some great women. But, just like most of us, there were some scoundrels. In every way Jesus became one of us, with a lineage like we have. He had the Dirty Uncle Sal who had embarrassed the family, the Aunt Drinky who flirted with all of the teenage boys and their fathers at family gatherings. He was not born in a palace surrounded by servants. Instead, there was no decent inn open for him. So he was born where the animals take shelter and eat. What humble beginnings for such a humble man! I think there is a great lesson there. Oh, Lord, help me be humble, in every way.

God is good, all the time.

December 18, 2008

If laughter is truly a medicine then I will have to go into rehab after this family vacation. I have been overdosing since the day we arrived.

We are staying in a beautiful log house right on Lake George. The view is gorgeous, the Adirondacks are breathtaking, the days are delightful and carefree (just like the tourist ads promise). The company is a riot. I have laughed so loud and so often that the pain in my chest seems minimal, compared the pain in my side. There have been a few times when I thought that I would not catch my breath, but I did, and then laughed some more.

Yesterday we celebrated Christmas. Happy moments started the day, and happy moments ended the day. Play-Doh, race cars, dinosaurs, Barbie, My Little Pony, Higgleytown Heroes, and puzzles dominated the scene. We had a blast watching the babies open the presents and play for hours. Fartsy the Snowman, complete with grape eyes, buttons smile, celery stalk nose, and ski cap sits as guard of the house. GG beat us at cards (or at least we told her she did). Turkey dinner with all of the fixings was served without the turkey. (Who knew that a frozen turkey would take so long!) In the end the kids decided which new toy they would sleep with and went upstairs for the night. With the fireplace crackling and snow softly falling, sleep came easy for all of us.

Today we are going to a place that has all kinds of fun things for the kids to play in and on; a climbing wall, a jumping area, and best of all, a pirate ship. For quite a while now Aurora has been convinced that Uncle Noah is a pirate. Crichton thinks that *he* is a pirate. Evayah and Cordelia don't really know what a pirate is, except that they saw one shaped like a cucumber in a Veggie Tales movie.

To be here, surrounded by God's creative beauty in nature and in people is awesome. So many things had to come together in perfect harmony for this time to take place. Two college schedules,   the   Navy's   timeline,   work   vacation   time, transportation, housing, all coming together for us. It was a Christmas miracle! Thank you, Lord.

God is good, all the time.

December 22, 2008

Glens Falls has a very nice hospital. Even though everyone who enters must go through a metal detector, the staff was very friendly and really knew their stuff.

I was in immense pain. The diagnosis was Trigeminal Neuralgia, or inflammation of the major nerve that runs like a branch on each side of a face. In my case the pain was on my right side from my forehead, down my eye, to my teeth, and ending at my neck. The good news is, the face pain made me forget about my other pain. I took Tegretol; Amanda used to take the same medicine to control her seizures. I think it is working because I cut back a bit on the Oxycodone. The end result is I am now even more fun when we play cards.

Since we have arrived in Lake George two feet of snow has fallen. Looking across the snow-covered lake over to the snow-splattered mountains is postcard perfect. I want to forever burn the picture in my memory; there is no way that it can be captured by Kodak. Every day we put more logs on the fire, watch the snow fall, play cards, and read our books. It's vacation Heaven. Thank you, Lord.

Some might wonder why I got yet another ailment, and on vacation of all things. Some sayings come to mind like "When it rains it pours" or "God won't give you more than you can handle" or "Isn't Steve sick and tired of taking Kim to the hospital?" The third one speaks the truth, but the first two I question. Sometimes it pours when it rains, but sometimes there is just a sprinkle. And I do not think that God gives you things like breast cancer and Trigeminal Neuralgia and crummy ovaries. God gives us things like peace, joy, and love. God is good and gives us good things. Unfortunately there is disease in the world. Disease does not discriminate. Disease chooses whomever it pleases and wreaks havoc on the victim and his or her family and friends.

That's when God comes in, a voice of reason in the chaos of pain. God brings solutions, wise doctors, medical breakthroughs, helpful medicine, peace that we cannot understand, joy where there should be none, love that wraps around us like a blanket. God is not the problem, God is the answer.

God is good, all the time.

December 26, 2008

After leaving behind the snow in the Adirondacks, it took an hour for Steve to locate and remove the snow from our parked car at the Grand Rapids airport. The car was left there by Noah and Susie. It's an Audi A6, so not a large car. After forty-six, yes, forty-six, inches of snow in the month of December (three times the West Michigan average) a car is buried. Fortunately the shuttle bus driver had pity on my husband who looked lost and forlorn, picked him up and drove him around until together they spotted a familiarly shaped mound so the snow removal could begin. The Christmas Spirit lives!

I thought that this was going to be a doctor free week. I was wrong. I had to go to my Primary Care office as a follow up to last week's hospital visit. Apparently the nerve issue in my face does not mend itself in a week. I need to stay on the medication for at least "months" according to Dr. Dibble. The worst part of the medication is it interacts badly with grapefruit. Grapefruit is right up there with mangos and tangerines for me. Now, not only is my diet already really restricted, but I cannot eat *grapefruit*. What's next, popcorn?

Today marks two weeks until my ovaries and uterus are removed. I have decided that I strongly dislike the word "hysterectomy." (I would say "hate" but the nuns at school would not allow us to use that word because it was such a strong term. We couldn't chew gum either. (Now I strongly dislike chewing gum.)

It sounds like an operation for older women. Plus the whole "bring on menopause" irks me. They say it like it is some joyful phrase, but it doesn't have the same ring as "bring on the competition" or "bring on the dessert."

I get emails telling me how great it will be to avoid using tampons each month, and that menopause is not that bad. Whatever. My family has not had happy menopause experiences. We are a little on the crazy side. As it is we all take "happy pills" just to avoid driving everyone around us nuts. If I get a little edgy, my kids check my supply of those special pills, and run to the all night pharmacy if necessary. Bring it on? Yeah, right.

I am not looking forward to "The Change" no matter how many uplifting emails I receive. I am considering getting my hair cut short, dying it fiery red and spiking it out with gel, just to reflect on the outside what I feel on the inside.

I need to quickly find a bunch of Dalmatians (101?) so that I can have a coat like Cruella Deville, and locate a long stem cigarette holder, like the one she held in the movie, but never lit. Stiletto heels used as a weapon will become part of my persona.

Oh dear, I'm on a downward spiral, aren't I? Okay then, happy thoughts! And let's change the subject.

The Christmas newspaper is always an interesting read. The state of the economy is reflected in the ad brochures, the recipes change from Christmas goodies to New Year's Eve appetizers, and the front page has an article about someone who did something good. Usually the front page is reserved for the worst crime or tragedy from the day before, but on Christmas the newspaper editors want us to feel happy. Thus an article, like this year's on Rev. Ed Dobson, fills the front page.

Rev. Dobson was the pastor of a very large church in Grand Rapids. He needed to step down when his Lou Gehrig's Disease (ALS) started affecting his job. But he has continued to be a great face of ministry in West Michigan and beyond. Rev. Dobson spent 2008 living like Jesus, a big challenge for anyone. The article was too short to really explain the depth of his transformation. I can't wait to read the book he wrote about his experience.

Why is it that we have to wait for Christmas day, or Saturday's Religion section to read about the good things that people are doing? I remember attending a sports banquet on the same night as the Oscars several years ago. I thought about the money and craziness that went into the actors' pat-on-the-back awards. Meanwhile, I was wearing my T.J. Maxx outfit, looking at the crèche paper decorations, all the while knowing the awards for the high school kids meant as much to them and their parents as the Oscars meant to the actors.

Yet, the next day the Oscar picks were mentioned on the front page as well as a few pages of the Entertainment section of the paper, and of course, the sports awards were not mentioned at all. Some of the sports banquet awardees were Chris Kaman, who now plays for the NBA, and mentions his faith in God in *Sports Illustrated* articles; Elissa Grochowalski, who spent several years helping babies from other countries find homes in the U.S. as she lived here and in Guatemala, and Micah Ophoff, who taught young students in Guatemala and led a church youth group with her husband, Anthony Verwys. Micah and Anthony also flew food and medicines into remote areas of the country.

Rob Dykstra was honored for bringing the love of Jesus to his financial planning office every day, and Kelly Hoeksema too. She went to school for nursing while helping her husband, Luke, through medical school. Luke's desire is to bring his faith to his job while working hard enough to support a couple of medical missionary trips each year.

There are many stories that come out of every sports banquet, graduation and awards assembly at every school. These stories do not make it to the front page of *The Grand Rapids Press*. These stories *do* make it to the eyes and ears of God. These are the stories that I love to hear and read about, but they are also the stories of humble people who don't need an award for what they are doing to help others. I praise God that Brad Pitt and Angelina Jolie are doing so much to help Katrina victims. I praise God for the many others I know who are doing the same thing, whose names and faces might remain anonymous here but will be heralded in Heaven. To those, thank you for all you do. Thanks for the time, talent, and treasure that you invest in helping our brothers and sisters. See you in Heaven.

God is good, all the time

December 29, 2008

This week's schedule goes something like this:

Monday: Doctor

Tuesday: Doctor

Wednesday: Avoid doctors at all costs and have a little champagne on New Year's Eve.

Thursday and Friday: Would be a visit to the doctor, however, in light of these days being holidays, my doctors are not working.

Meanwhile, my face feels better though I have grown a bit weary of the old joke, "Yeah, but it's *killin' me!*" The blobs of flesh and expander on my chest, however, continue to hurt, though not as bad or as often as they used to, but they hurt nonetheless.

Today, I am to be cleared for the January 9 surgery. Tomorrow I will be scheduled for the expander removal/permanent replacement surgery. I am wondering if I get to keep the expanders like the way a kid will keep a tooth. Maybe there is an Expander Fairy that will bring me money in the night. Maybe I should make artwork out of them and hang them over my fireplace. Maybe I should just let the doctor throw them away, never to hurt anyone again. I think that tomorrow I also get to choose the new ones. In the past my sister-in-law and daughter-in-law have taken me to the appointments that Steve is unable to attend. But this one might require a husband's presence. I will find out if he and his wisdom are available.

I have two confessions. (I grew up Catholic and right now there's not a priest in sight.) First of all, I had a piece of fudge and three cookies on Christmas Day. Sugar! Real Sugar! But please understand that Andi uses real vanilla from the Dominican Republic in her fudge, the best vanilla in the world. And the cookies, well, those were really good, melt-in-your-mouth lemon cookies that Renee makes every year. I *know*—no excuses. But it was Christmas Day, and I have been really good. I will say the assigned number of Our Father's and Hail Mary's.

Secondly, I am jealous of New Year's Celebrations. Yes, jealousy, the Green-Eyed Monster. I wish I could celebrate, and I'm bummed about the New Year, so I'm jealous. Somehow in God's divine plan, we get a new start every 365 days. No matter how we have failed, or the world has failed us, once a year we get to put it all behind and start anew. It's a fresh beginning, a new day with new promises and new hope. That is why we stay up until midnight on New Year's Eve and watch the big ball drop, because we want to know that nothing else crummy is going to happen this year, and we want to celebrate the first few precious, unscarred moments of the New Year.

Some historian came up with the concept of the New Year's Baby. Can't you just picture that sweet little baby, full of hope and wonderment, cooing and giggling? But somehow by the end of the year the picture turns into Father Time, sporting a long gray beard, a huge clock around his neck like Flava Flav, and a somewhat sinister smile. Depending on how 2008 treated you, Father Time could be laughing with you or at you. It is amazing what happens to that New Year's Baby's anticipation in one year.

For those who have had a rough year and want to begin again, praise God and move on. Leave it behind. Move ahead. Turn your ship in a new direction.

I have a good friend who really needs to celebrate leaving the old year behind her. In 2008, she helped a young nephew with cancer see that Heaven is really full of wonder, and now he is there, enjoying the wonder. She also helped her niece learn about God's love, and then her niece died on Christmas Day, released from this earth to experience God's love in a new way. Others close to her have also left this world.

She sacrificed all of 2008 for other people. She needs to not only have champagne at the end of this year, but she needs to stay up long enough to bring in the next year. She needs to go outside before midnight and scream from the top of her lungs "I am mad as H-E-Double Toothpicks, and I am not going to take it anymore!" Then after midnight, she needs to fall on her knees and praise God for a New Year, and with it new hope, new joy, new beginning.

This year Father Time has been a bit harsh with me. I have two surgeries ahead, with one surgery behind. As much as I want to be a glass-half-full person, today it is just not happening. I want to celebrate the New Year (although I have to admit that staying up until midnight sounds less appealing each year. Does the ball dropping have the same effect if you watch it on TiVo at 9 a.m. the next morning?).

But I still want that feeling, that awesome anticipation of a new beginning, wiping the slate clean and starting all over again. I don't begrudge the celebrators just the celebration. I want it for me. I want it for my friend whose daughter might be spending New Years Eve at DeVos Children's Hospital instead of at home where kids should be, drinking sparkling grape juice, and getting potato chips all over the couch. I want it for my friend who is the toughest brain cancer patient ever. I want it for her family. I want it for my friend who has just gone through Christmas without her husband. I want it for my husband who has put his medical issues on hold while I get through mine. I want it for me.

God is the God of new beginnings. He is the one who wipes the slate clean and gives us a fresh start. He is the foundation of hope, the cornerstone of joy, the rock where newness begins. I thank God in my heart and in my head that I know this truth. I praise God for who He is. When I raise that glass of sugar-free, non-alcoholic champagne (fruit juice) on New Year's Eve, I will toast an amazing God, and a new start for all of us. Here is hoping that your toast will be the same.

God is good, all the time.

December 31, 2008

My appointment with Dr. 90210-49503 did not go as expected. I thought he was going to tell me how great everything looked, show me some samples, and schedule a date for surgery. Instead he injected more saline, expanding another 60ccs which I believe puts me at about 550ccs on each side.

According to an online conversion table, I am now carrying 4.649428122 cups of liquid on my chest. That translates to about 2.4 pounds, or better, a "C." This is one area of life that getting a "C" is better than an "A" or a "B." Since I have been a "D," or more since about fourth grade, "C" sounds pretty good.

I have to go back in about three weeks to talk about another surgery.

Yes, I am very sore. It hurts! I feel like my breasts start at the very center of my chest and wrap themselves under and around my armpits. My arms cannot hang freely at my sides, as if I have just finished sweating through an hour of bench pressing. Pills are good. Driving is bad with pills. Lots of things are bad with pills, but I would rather have pills than pain. Dr. 90210-49503 would call the pain "discomfort." My Dad would call the pain "a good offer upper" (Catholic lingo). The Kingston Trio would call the pain, "Mariah." I call the pain lots of names, some of which are better left unwritten.

Steve's mom lost her brother, John, this week. He wandered away into Heaven. He had been ill, and was getting worse. His pain and suffering is no longer, but his family's pain has just begun. Life has a funny way of doing that, exchanging one pain for another. It is kind of like the old joke when the patient says, "Hey Doc, my elbow is killing me," so the doctor hits him in the stomach so he can forget about his elbow. That is what it feels like sometimes, a punch in the gut. A diagnosis, a death, a divorce, a car accident—they're all punches in the gut. There are not enough Tums at Walgreens to take that pain away. It takes time. Time really is the great healer.

I remember going to Meijer to pick something up within a day or two of my mom dying. I looked around and was amazed at what I saw. People were shopping, looking at magazines, picking up crying babies, talking to friends, all as if nothing had happened.

It was the same when I was told I had cancer. Life just went on. It did not wait for me to mourn. It just kept going. It did not matter that I wanted it to stop. I needed it to stop. I needed everyone to know what just happened to me. But there is no special parking spot for "Mourning Daughter" or "Cancer

Patient." Life went on, and eventually so did I. Today does not feel the same as the day that I was diagnosed. I have a lot of the same feelings, but it does not feel the same. Time teaches you things like how to live when someone you love is not there. Time lessens the pain without erasing the memories. Six months from now, things will be better for Aunt Margie, and in two years, things will be better yet. Old Father Time, our pal, keeps marching on.

Tonight time will click away. One hour until midnight. Ten minutes until midnight. One minute until midnight. Ten seconds, nine, eight, seven, six, five, four, three, two, one! Happy New Year Everyone! May God bring blessings, joy and love untold into the New Year for all of us.

God is good, all the time.

January 2, 2009

Pain is still my constant companion, but now my cup is running over. The self-pity that I felt before the end of 2008 left with the dawn of a new year. January 1 really does bring new optimism and new hope. Even though I am very cold and cannot feel my toes, I am thinking things are looking up. Gas prices are down, the snow has made everything clean again, Dick Clark counted down the New Year without a single wrinkle, and I am just a week away from cramp-free living. Life does not get much better than this.

God is good. I remember that most of the time. Sometimes He reminds me. Sometimes the reminders are gentle nudges, and sometimes more like a two-by-four to the temple. Today I had a great two-by-four experience.

My dad invited me to lunch with Father Jose from St. Francis Catholic Church, a church near Burton and Division. St. Francis was home to Steve for many years. The tree he climbed to get out of class is still there, as is the spot where he put the pinching beetle down the back of the girl with the back brace. He can still picture the air under the feet of the classmate who was raised up by his ears after upsetting a lay teacher. I am sure that there are still burn marks on the concrete walls from the different chemicals mixed together by Sister Susan Duffy, who had a passion for chemistry, and taught Steve more in seventh grade than he learned in high school. For a lot of years St. Francis was home to kids, nuns and lay teachers. Now the school is empty, Father Jose says Mass in both English and Spanish each week, and Steve would be hard pressed to find anyone he recognized from the old days.

After an incredible Mass and celebration of Jesus on December 23, Father Jose retired to the house that the church provides. In the night he heard rain and hoped it wouldn't cause flooding. In the early morning he suddenly heard the fire alarm. Father Jose went across the hall to find a broken radiator spewing steam, which initiated the rain from the sprinkler system. The water ran down to the first floor and basement, soaking through the ceiling and walls. All of the old plaster, pictures, furniture, and light fixtures were destroyed.

The dining room which held his mother's beautifully carved table, chairs and china cabinet had water pouring in from the center light fixture. Precious mementos from his home in Mexico, as well as treasured items that had held a place in the rectory for many years were reduced to rubble on the warped hardwood floors. The insurance company sent a cleaning and construction company and let Father know that they would also pay for a hotel room until he was able to get back into his house.

Christmas Eve in a hotel did not sound appealing, so after celebrating an extra special Midnight Mass he returned home to the one room that was not damaged by the water, the living room. Ready to start a fire and bask in the glow of Christmas spirit, he entered the room only to discover that the Christmas tree had fallen over. Deciding to leave and take the Christmas spirit with him, he discovered that the door would not open. He was alone in the middle of the night, Christmas morning, in a broken house, with a broken tree and a broken door.

St. Francis is not what it used to be. Tithes are smaller and the building is older. As nuns stopped teaching, tuition prices increased, so student population decreased, and eventually the school was shut down. Building maintenance is a big job, and paying bills is an even bigger job. A broken pipe going to the boiler system is making a rusty ice rink at the north end of the parking lot, and it cannot be repaired until next Tuesday.

Although one classroom is being used for classes to teach Somali refugees English, and another is used by a psychologist who offers free counseling once each week, the small token the tenants pay does not cover heat and electricity. There may have been a day at St. Francis when a boardroom of people would gather to discuss what to do with the excess monies. Now the meetings are probably much like when I was on the board of a Christian School, with no such thing as excess funds.

I attended Mass there in the small chapel at the church. Father Jose read the pre-chosen words from the Book of John, spoken by John the Baptist. A group of people asked John the Baptist who he was, and he told them that he is the guy paving the way for Jesus to come. John the Baptizer went on to tell them he was baptizing them with water, but that Jesus would anoint them with the Holy Spirit, God.

Before the service Father Jose asked if he could anoint me with oil and pray for my health and my upcoming surgery. When Father called me up near the end of Mass, the other five attendees (six with God) followed, placed their hands on me and prayed. John anointed with water, Jesus with the Holy Spirit, and Father Jose with oil, anointing, dedicating to God.

In between Mass and lunch, I saw just the damages on the first floor of Father Jose's house. I saw the area after the fallen plaster and other debris was removed, and the rooms swept clean. Still, the job ahead would be daunting: drywall, primer, paint, molding, window treatments, flooring, on and on. The money needed to clean it all up and make the needed repairs, not to mention really make a difference in the lives of his parishioners, is a large dollar amount. Yet, the spirit and the heart of Father Jose reflected solutions, not problems, joy not sorrow, and love not hate.

Father Jose has given himself completely to help people. Not just on Sundays, or on a missions trip, or in an update, but every day, all day.

Father Jose is truly dedicated to God, doing amazing things, helping lots of people. Yet, the boiler pipe is broken, a radiator busted, heirloom furniture is ruined, and the Christmas tree fell over. He's one hundred percent sold out for Jesus, but still dealing with the crap that happens in life. We all do. We all have crap. Billy Graham has crap and so does Bill Gates. My crap is not nearly as bad as a lot of the crap out there. Father Jose knows people who are losing their homes, others do not have money for groceries this week, and some have lost their jobs and need to move to another state or back to Mexico to find work.

As I walked into my five bedroom house in the suburbs, I thanked God for Father Jose, whom he used as a two-by-four in my life. I have got it made here. My house is warm, my bed is warmer. In one week I will say goodbye to cramps, P.M.S. and tampons. (Well, it won't be called P.M.S. anymore.) In a few weeks I get to pick out the beautiful, tear drop implants and a great tattoo color. I get to eat yummy things like oranges, scrambled eggs with creamed cheese, mangos and carrots. Shoot, I can even eat sugar-free chocolate, which can be as good as the real sugar stuff. Steve lets me use him as a hot water bottle for my ice cold feet at night. My car has heaters in the seat. I can read. I can type almost as fast as I can think. I have great friends, great family, and great slippers. My cup is truly overflowing.

God is good, all the time.

January 6, 2008

The pain is a bit better but, for some reason, I slept for twelve hours last night. I fell asleep watching TV (the premier of "The Bachelor," featuring a nice single guy with a cute little boy, and twenty-five women all looking for love. It's totally unrealistic, but interesting to watch). I woke up long enough to brush my teeth and crawl into bed. I didn't wake up until 9:00 a.m. this morning. I think the medicine I take to make my face not hurt (quit with the jokes already) is making me really tired. So, now that I have achieved my doctorate in self-diagnosis and prescription analysis, my plan is to cut back on that medication to see if the pain still stays away and find out if I have more energy. Hopefully, it will work. Meanwhile, if you need any medical advice my shingle is hanging on the door.

I spent Sunday afternoon reminiscing about my mom, Aunt Maggie, and Uncle Chuck, with a few of my cousins, a couple of sisters-in-law, and an aunt. There is such a freedom in speech when there are only women in a room. Laughter comes as easy as tears, and more often. The stories told require no gender censorship. Dreams are discussed, both the sleeping kind and the daytime kind. Old husbands, old boyfriends, and old dogs all get their fair share of conversation.

We looked at pictures of happy moments, of weddings, Christmas parties, vacations, and golf outings. But some of the happy moments brought sadness with them; some marriages are no more, families have drifted apart, people we loved now gone. Some pictures seem like they were taken just yesterday, while others spark a memory long forgotten. Some things we are glad to leave in the past like afro perms and mullets. Other things we wish that we could relive just one more time, just one more day. If we could just start over, wouldn't it be wonderful? If we just knew then what we know now, wouldn't things have turned out differently?

Like Sister Mary Louise used to say: "If 'ifs' and 'buts' were candy and nuts, we'd all have a box of chocolates." But then life turns into Forrest Gump's Mom's idea of never knowing what you're going to get. Some of life is pretty predictable, such as water coming out of the shower when turned on, the sun rising, hunger happening two hours after eating Chinese food, and junk mail coming every day. But it is the unpredictable things that shift our lives in unexpected ways, such as losing a job, divorce, a move, death, and disease.

I remember when my dad lost his job in 1979. He had made a good living at a business that he started and then sold but still supervised. Running that company is what my dad did, it was a big part of who he was, or so I thought. I soon found out that it was not the job that made the man. It was barely a bump in the road for him. He just found another opportunity and started a new business that ended up being much more successful than the last. He just kept going. There was no "woe is me" time for him, he just got back on that horse and rode. My dad had faith that God would take care of him, and his faith brought him through. My dad may have doubted himself for a second, but he never doubted God.

I hope that when all of this medical stuff is over, my kids will think the same of me. I hope they see my faith and my unwavering trust in God. I hope they understand that without the Lord, I would be scared and unsure of what may happen next. Instead I know that God is by my side right now and always. That He will not leave me. God will be there on Friday to hold my hand just like He did on October 21. I hope that they recognize that faith is my foundation for strength. *I hope that they know that . . .*

God is good, all the time.

Surgery Eve
January 8, 2009

By this time tomorrow I should be in a deep sleep, with my colonoscopy behind me, and my ovaries on their way out. After checking in at 5:30 a.m. tomorrow morning, surgery is due to begin at 7:30 a.m. Today I can eat food until noon and then begin the bowel prep, which involves clear liquids, Flagyl and all. Besides a couple of bouts with the flu, I don't know that I have ever had a colonoscopy-worthy colon. When Steve had his about a year ago, Dr. Ahzeem was very specific on preparing perfectly so that no tiny morsel could lead to a misdiagnosis. I, too, will fall under the harsh judgment of the Great Butt Doctor and hope that I can live up to his strict standards. Steve really struggled with his prep and did everything by the book. His rating from Dr. Behind was 8 out of 10. I am hoping to beat that score. Clean bowel, here I come!

Today I am a bit anxious about tomorrow. I don't know that surgery is something I would ever get excited about. Even if it was to get rid of crow's feet, give me a Brazilian butt lift or some much needed liposuction, I might be excited for the results but not excited for the procedure. I am sure that waking up tomorrow will be easier than waking up after the last surgery. I am hoping that the pain of the five small incisions in my stomach (including the one forever hidden in my navel), will not compare to the pain of removing what once fed my babies. (I didn't really feed them that way. I tried with Noah, almost starved him, and I switched to formula. Apparently size and milk quantity do not go hand in hand.)

Webster defines anxious as "greatly worried." Most of the time God uses the word to tell us not to be anxious. Like when He says not to be worried about tomorrow because tomorrow has enough worry of its own. Or not to be anxious about what you will eat or what you will wear because life, living, is so much more than food, and the body is so much more than clothes. And what about the flowers and the birds; God takes care of them but how much more does He love us? He will take care of us.

My favorite reference right now is when Paul told the Philippians not to be anxious about anything (even surgery), but let God know what you need and be thankful for what you

CRY UNTIL YOU LAUGH

have. Today that is what I am doing. Today I am thankful for sugar-free Jell-O, popsicles, white grape juice, and chicken broth. I am thankful for no more monthly cramps and no more tampons. I am thankful for clean drinking water and clear ice cubes. I am thankful for indoor plumbing and soft toilet paper. I am thankful for a Walgreens on every corner and the pharmacist that works there. I am thankful for the flavor of magnesium citrate and pills that can be swallowed. I am thankful for clean hospitals and great doctors. I am thankful for pain pills and laxatives. I am thankful for health insurance and the job that provides it. I am thankful for medical research and those that fund it. I am thankful for God who loves me and whom I love back. I am thankful that God listens to prayers and that I have friends who pray. I am thankful that tomorrow I begin my recovery, and for clean sheets to recover on.

God is good, all the time.

Post-Surgery
January 13, 2009

I have now officially crossed over to the "Women without Ovaries" club. I think red hats are supposed to lure me into boutiques now. When I'm able to go shopping again, I will see what happens.

"Surgery was a bitch," said Dr. McAnalogy. Apparently it took twice as long as a "normal hysterectomy." My uterus was "super glued" to my bladder, which took a full hour to separate. He found a polyp in my bladder, which precipitated the need for a surgical urologist to come in and assist. There was also some stuff that Dr. McAnalogy took pictures of that Steve had seen only four times before in "Alien," "Aliens," "Alien 3" and "Alien Resurrection." Paul had seen it in "Ghost Busters." Dr. McAnalogy said that he had seen it before, not often, but maybe once or twice. When it was all said and done, a few extra doctors visited the Surgery Room, I was under much longer than expected, there are four cuts healing on my stomach, and the pathologists have plenty of work ahead of them.

I did win the clean colon contest! Put up one for the home team! Steve was disappointed, but he should be used to it, because I try to beat him at everything. Contests are my thing, and actually, they are a family thing. As a kid I couldn't walk to the mailbox without it turning into a race. Even as an adult, my father and I would compete at anything, it didn't matter if it was a flight of stairs, a long hallway or a swim across a pool, the race was on. I come by competitiveness naturally, which is why I enjoyed competing in sports and coaching. Winning is good. Steve does beat me in tennis, but I have the victoriously clean colon. I would say that colon trumps tennis any day.

In most every competition there is just one happy person or team in the end. Leading up to the championship, teams might say, "if we just make it to quarterfinals," or "if we just make it to the finals," then we will be happy. Reality is that nobody is happy except the final winners, the first place team. Everyone else walks away shaking their heads, wondering what they could have done differently. Meanwhile the winners celebrate.

Of course, much of life is that not mimicked by sports; life doesn't always have a win or lose paradigm. The choices we make, the dedication we put into something, the love we give, and how hard we fight all help to determine whether we will win or lose. I choose to win. I choose to fight and overcome. I choose to love and give and believe. Like the old song says, "The victory is mine when the battle is the Lord's."

God is good, all the time.

January 15, 2009

I have definitely developed a prejudice when it comes to doctors. I want them to be my age or younger. When the anesthesiologist walked in with his white mane and wrinkles reflecting my father's age, all I could picture was going into surgery and being handed a bottle of whiskey and a bullet to bite on.

Then my imagination went further: the bullet would do great injury to my teeth so I would have to go to Fred the Dentist. I love Fred but I am not fond of the dentist side of him, or anyone's dentist side for that matter. The sunny side of going to Fred's office would be to see his wife and my good friend, Joyce. I would make Joyce promise that she would talk during the whole dental procedure. Of course, Fred's hands in my mouth would make talking for me difficult (but not impossible, I can talk under pretty much any circumstances). But Joyce could talk to Fred and I could listen and try to be distracted from the drilling and sucking and more drilling. Fred and Joyce are both very funny. Listening to them during a dental visit almost makes the dental visit worthwhile. They could really take their show on the road, which they do from time to time. But the road to them is third world countries in areas where dental care is non-existent and pulling a bad tooth means saving a life. I have been with them in third world countries, and they are still funny. Fortunately they both know some Spanish (especially Joyce). I have heard Fred ask for the "Proximo

Potato" or something like that. Joyce, on the other hand, can show people the love of Jesus with her smile and a few words that they and she understands.

Man, I can digress when not wanting to think about surgery! Anyway, so the guy was older than I would have liked. They just assign you an anesthesiologist, your name goes on the board, and a doctor is randomly selected for you. You do not get to research and find the best one. You don't get to ask the nurses who they like. You just have to trust that who they give you will be good, and then pay him or her when the bill comes in. And the bill is like the price of a new car. Who would buy a new car without looking at "Car and Driver" for all of the specs on which is best?

Digressing.

Focus.

So, I didn't get to pick the grizzled old doctor, and in the end, I still would have liked someone else. The drugs he administered took a long time to leave my system, which was a much different experience than my last surgery. The recovery nurse was never able to wake me up in recovery, so I was taken to my room after a couple of hours. And I was puffy—really puffy. Like the Michelin Man or The Rock on "The Fantastic Four" puffy. I am still a bit on the puffy side.

My hands are sore. I am not sure why, but I blame the older doctor. Another thing: he gave me anti-nervous stuff before I was wheeled down to the big, sterile, scary room, probably so when I got there I wouldn't jump off the table and run the other way. That part was alright, but then in the scary room he didn't have me count backwards from 100, or name every farm animal, or think about drinking a Pina Colada while sitting on the beach listening to the waves splashing against the rocks. Instead someone said "Put your right leg here. Give me your left arm. Your left leg needs to go there . . . ."

I confess, I am right/left impaired. It is a handicap I try to keep in the closet. I can do north/south/east/west. I have even mastered a.m. and p.m. (a.m. *should* be afternoon because it starts with "a," but it doesn't). But I think that I had Chicken Pox during right/left day in kindergarten, and ever since then my mind just does not function properly. So there I was, drugged, giving them maybe the right leg, maybe the wrong arm, and the next thing I knew I was in a hospital room, suffering severe cotton mouth and wondering why I was having back labor. For all I knew the doctor took advantage of me, I slept for nine months, and now was delivering a big baby that was lying on my spine. No one warned me about back pain. It was and remains pretty intense.

Digressing.

Refocus.

All that to say, I believe that the system should change and everyone should have the right to choose the doctor who will be controlling whether they live or die on an operating room table. I still have pretty bad back pain, like back labor or really bad back cramps that some of us get monthly. Steve bought the most expensive heating pad that money can buy at Walgreens for $35. It helps quite a bit but is cumbersome to move from chair to bed to computer chair to recliner to bed. Right now the heating pad and I are pretty inseparable.

Other parts of me are not giving off good vibes either. I think while the old doctor had me under, Dr. McAnalogy took a baseball bat to my stomach, because bruises are starting to appear (I think that I have my proof). I watch the clock when it is getting to be time to take another pain pill. The pills help, just not entirely.

I have been told I will feel "much better" when I am a week out from the surgery. I am looking forward to waking up Saturday morning feeling "much better." Because my surgery became so extensive, the two week recovery turned into six weeks. Basically that means that I cannot lift anything over twenty pounds for that amount of time. The only time I lift over twenty pounds is when I rearrange furniture or lift up one of my grandchildren. I think I can forgo spring cleaning for six weeks, but the baby lifting will be hard to forego.

Next week I have an appointment with Dr. 90210-49503 to schedule the next surgery. I am not sure how much time they will give me to recover from this one, but it will be nice to have all surgical procedures behind me. I am also not sure that choosing a tattoo color while under the influence of pain medication is a good idea or maybe it is . . . hmm. Next week I will also see Dr. McAnalogy. Hopefully he will have some test results and we can all celebrate.

I watched Rob Bell's "Everything is Spiritual" DVD the other day. (I would highly recommend it!) Rob has so many factoids in his brain at any one time. In the DVD, he talks about how God started with creating and seven days later rested. When people have been enslaved at different times throughout history, work would be seven days a week with no rest. People would forget, or simply not know how to be human and how to rest. Even now there seems to be a medal for workaholics who work lots of hours, seven days a week. (Really any word that ends in "aholics" should be given counseling, not a medal.)

Resting is good. It is alright to rest, whatever that means to you. To me, resting is lying on the couch with Steve watching a football game on a Sunday afternoon. It can be playing cards with Amanda, watching the past seasons of "Grey's Anatomy" with Susie, or going out to dinner with friends. Resting for me is also that happy moment when the babies are over, and it is "cuddle time." *Resting*. It can mean whatever it means to you. It is important to do. Lately, I have been getting really good at resting. Maybe I am making up for all those years when resting eluded me. I am getting so good at it I think I will make it part of my weekly routine, after all of this is over. I hope you find rest.

God is good, all the time.

January 16, 2009

"When it rains it pours," my friend said recently. I, of course, tried to find a silver lining. "It doesn't always pour when it rains, sometimes it just drizzles," I said, cheerfully. "Plus you get that beautiful rainbow at the end."

Well, tonight it's definitely pouring and I am so ready for that rainbow. We found out today that it's Steve who may be in trouble, health wise, when all this time we thought it was me.

Steve had been having stomach troubles since the day that I was diagnosed with cancer. Of course, his primary care physician, as well as a gastrointestinal specialist, blamed the aches on anxiety. Today he was in pain and drove himself to the emergency room since I am still in recovery mode. After an ultrasound, some blood work, and a CAT scan, he was admitted. The tests revealed a large mass (I hate that word unless it is used in reference to a Catholic service) on his liver. Tomorrow morning we will meet with a radiologist and a surgical oncologist. The plan is to perform a biopsy as soon as possible.

Please pray. Right now I am a little miffed at God. Yeah, I know, He did not give this mass to Steve, whatever it is. But anger is the emotion I am choosing right now. Maybe I am not really mad at God but just mad in general. My stomach hurts, my back hurts, my chest hurts, and now my heart is killing me.

Steve is *the one*. He is the one I am supposed to grow old with. He is the one who will tell me if there is ketchup on my face, who says "No honey" when I ask him if something makes me look fat. He is the one who scratches my back in the places that I can't reach (short arms run in my family). His shoulder is exactly the right size for my head. We fit together perfectly when we spoon. Steve is the one, my always and forever. *Please* pray.

God is good, all the time (really).

January 18, 2008

Remember this old joke?

> "I've got some good news and some bad news. Which do you want first?"
>
> "The good news is you look just like your mother."
>
> "The bad news is your mother is ugly."

Just like the old joke, this update has some good news and some bad news.

The good news is that all the stuff Dr. McAnalogy took out of my body was benign. I am cancer free and proud of it. I am on day two of antibiotics for a UTI (urinary tract infection for you healthy, non-medical people), so I feel really great. The next step is to get my beautiful new implants. A really good friend of mine said that she saw a tee shirt that read "Yes they are fake, my other ones tried to kill me." I think I will skip the tee shirt and just let people wonder because they will be fabulous.

The bad news: things are not looking great right now for Steve. Some blood work came back this morning and the results were discouraging. There are various blood tests that measure cancer tumor markers. One is "CA 19-9," which has a normal range of 0-40. Steve's came back at 169,998 (yes, that is almost 170,000). There is another one called "CEA," which has a normal range of 0-2.5, and Steve's number is 82.5.

These results, combined with the CAT scan readings, are making the doctors assume that Steve has a very aggressive, nasty cancer. The CAT scan shows what they believe to be cancer in not only his liver, but also the fatty layer of whatever it is that protects the stomach and his colon.

Tomorrow at 10:00 am Dr. Meisner will perform a colonoscopy. ("Perform" is an interesting word choice, like it's some kind of theatrical presentation.) Sometime after that, the radiologist will perform a biopsy.

As I write this, I am in a canoe paddling down the river Denial. I am hoping and praying the old adage is true: "Don't assume anything because it just makes an ass out of u and me." That's exactly what the doctors are doing, but they can't know for sure until the colonoscopy and biopsy are done and tested. My strongest desire is that the doctors tell us he just has an infection or something and that everything will be just fine.

In The Message translation of the Bible, 1 Corinthians 13:13 reads, "Trust steadily in God, hope unswervingly, love extravagantly. And the best of the three is love." Faith, hope and love—that's what we are supposed to do. I *trust* that God will hold on to us tightly, *hope* that God will celebrate in our victory, and *love* Steve with every ounce of my being.

God is good, all the time.

January 21, 2009

Love is an interesting, multi-faceted, ever changing emotion. Love brings into our lives the highest of highs, the lowest of lows, and everything in between. Little compares to the overwhelming love felt speaking wedding vows, or the first time you look into your newborn's eyes. And little compares to the broken heart of a lost love, or a child that has wondered away. Sometimes love is not high or low but both.

We do not yet have a diagnosis on Steve. He was discharged from the hospital yesterday, just as I was being admitted to treat a kidney infection. Praise God I am home today. This afternoon Steve and I are meeting with Dr. Chung, surgical oncologist. Hopefully by then the pathology report from Monday's liver biopsy will be explained to us. Until then, I am still praying that all of the doctors are wrong, and that Steve does not have cancer and will be treated for an infection that will require warm weather, sunshine, beach sand, and antibiotics to heal.

I have been in love with Steve for most of the time I have known him. I am talking *in love*, not just love, not like, but that butterflies-in-the-stomach, can't-wait-to-see-him, forgiving-of-morning-breath kind of *in love*. Now, I have been punched in the gut by love, dragged down, beaten, with my heart torn out and stomped on. I have the high love, the low love, not one or the other but both.

Fortunately God knows about love. In fact, He came up with the concept. Love is really great, but it can really hurt. Right now it is great and it hurts—so much.

God is good, all the time.

Second Addition

January 21, 2009

Jesus is referred to as a "rock" in the Bible a few times: The Rock of salvation, Cornerstone, and the Rock of Israel are just a few of the references. Steve is also a rock, his faith unwavering, his love non-discriminate, his hope unrelenting.

Today Steve and I found out that the liver biopsy was positive for Adeno-Carcinoma. Although the doctors don't know the extent of the cancer, they do know it's *not* the cancer they wished they would have found. This is a fast growing, highly aggressive cancer that could easily take his life within the next year. On Friday we are going to speak with an oncologist to talk about chemotherapy options that could possibly shrink the tumors.

I am not a "name it, claim it" person. I do not believe that saying the "C" word makes cancer hang on. Cancer is not that smart. All cancer knows is that it wants to grow more cancer. I also do not believe that Steve has cancer because of sin or some unresolved issue in his life, or that praying a certain prayer spoken a certain way cures someone.

I do believe prayer and asking God for healing can bring about healing, it just doesn't have to be prayed using certain words. When God was walking around in the form of Jesus, He turned blind eyes into seeing eyes, bad limbs into walking limbs, unhearing ears into hearing ears, and more. God is still here with us every day. It's just that now, we see Him more clearly in some situations than others. Sometimes He still heals, even cancer.

This is our prayer, that Steve would receive a complete healing from the same God that fed a crowd of people with just a couple of loaves of bread and a few fish.

God is good, all the time.

January 22, 2009

I now know what it is to be in shock, and I don't like it. Every part of my body is numb, my head, my hands, my heart. My head can't focus, my hands are trembling, and my heart can't feel. Right now my house could literally fall in around me, and I don't think that I would care, and perhaps not even notice. I try to focus, to feel, but all I want to do is lie down next to Steve. I go from crying to not crying to crying again. I am the closest one that can help Steve, but right now I am helpless. I have a pit in my stomach the size of the New Hampshire; I am trying to blame it on my kidney infection. I have no energy, no appetite and I haven't washed my hair in a couple of days. I'm shell shocked.

This morning around 3 a.m., I was praying and thinking. I wondered why it is that when we know God has this great vacation spot ready for us, better than any Caribbean Island, European Tour, even better than Disney World, why do we fight death? Why do we struggle so hard and wage war against a disease that wants so badly to take our life and send us to Heaven? Why the battle? I have seen people who fought so hard they failed to live the life they had left.

Please understand, Steve and I will fight this cancer crap until God tells Steve to fight no more. But while fighting, I pray that we also live so that we are aware of God's desires for us.

One day at a time, life will continue to happen. Every day our prayer will be that good comes from such an ugly thing.

Lord, please heal my husband just like you have brought miraculous healing to others. Please let good things happen during this trial. Please give us wisdom in dealing with all the medical and non-medical stuff in our lives. Help us to live, really live, each day we have and count each day a blessing from you. I love you.

God is good, all the time.

January 23, 2009

Steve wins. The competition is over. It no longer matters that I won the clean colon contest or 102 hands of Rummy to his 99. He wins and that is okay with me.

Today Steve and I met with Dr. Brinker, a wonderful oncologist. He spent a couple of hours with us explaining the diagnosis, deciphering the test results, and deciding the plan of attack. The doctor received additional information regarding the liver biopsy from the pathology lab. Steve's cancer either started in the pancreas or the bile ducts, and either way it is Stage Four (which means it has traveled, landed and grown extensively in his abdomen), ductal (as in, it started in the ducts, which is bad news), and non-operable and incurable.

If Steve chooses not to have any chemotherapy he would live on earth another four-six months. The average person with this type of cancer will live about one year with chemo treatments.

Steve is anything but average. He is a fifty-one-year-old, fit, thin, non-smoking, non-drinking, non-recreational drug using handsome guy. With Steve, one year could turn into two or more. With God, one year could turn into fifty.

So Steve wins. If God gives Steve an incredible medical miracle we will celebrate like its 1999. If God carries Steve to paradise, we will celebrate like crazy as well.

On Wednesday Steve will begin chemo. He will be on a twenty-one day cycle with two weeks on and one week off. Two different chemo drugs will be attacking those nasty cancer cells in two different ways, one by pill and the other through I.V. He will take a couple of pills every day for 14 days and have I.V. chemo on Day One and Day Eight. After two cycles another CAT Scan will be done to see how the cancer is responding. Shrinking the tumors will help with his pain. The side effects are supposed to be minimal so I should still be able to run my fingers through his gorgeous hair.

Every day right now is a gift. Every moment, every joke, every prayer, every kiss from a grandchild is more precious than it used to be. This is really the way Steve and I should have been living all along. Right there in black and white is a verse we have read many times, telling us to live each day to the fullest because we do not know what tomorrow will bring. I failed at understanding what living that way meant before. Now I think I know. I believe it means to not live in the future wondering what life will be like in March or July or next Christmas, but instead enjoy today seeing what newness it holds. Every day is different than the one before and the ones that will come later. Today is the day that we will focus on. Today we will enjoy the gift, open the beautiful wrapping and be surprised by the contents.

God is good, all the time.

January 24, 2009

This "one day at a time" thing is really working. It is amazing — when you forget about the future, daily life somehow has more meaning. Things with God are so backwards. I'm talking about how we are supposed to have the faith of a child instead of an old guy. I would think that the old guy would have more faith, but a child's faith is so innocent, unwavering, and complete.

Complete. That's the word God gave Steve yesterday morning before the oncologist appointment. Steve is complete. I think that over the next several months, Steve will learn everything God means by that. Right now it is a comfort, a warm, fuzzy blanket, a special word from God.

Other God-things seem backwards too. Who sends peace in the middle of a storm? Someone might throw a life jacket, maybe, but not peace that wraps around you so that the storm blows all around but never gets close enough to muss your hair. Then there's hope. Why is there hope when doctors throw around terms like "terminal," and tell us they can "treat" Steve but not "cure" him? Most of the time I expect God to come through the front door, but He is quietly entering through the back door. I don't know if I will ever understand the way God chooses to do things, but I have to say He is genius.

My son Noah quoted a story to me this morning:

A farmer has a horse. The horse goes missing. His neighbor says, "I am so sorry about your horse." The farmer replies, "Who knows what is right or wrong." The horse returns with many more horses following him. The farmer's son rides one of the new horses, falls off and breaks his leg. The neighbor says, "I am so sorry about your son." The farmer replies, "Who knows what is right or wrong." Soon after, the military comes looking for young men to go fight in the war. They bypass the farmer's son because of his broken leg. The neighbor says, "I am so glad that your son did not have to face war." The farmer replies, "Who knows what is right or wrong."

God does what God does. In this backwards world I would want Steve to stay here as long as possible, but I also do not want to see him suffer. Plus, I am so excited for him to go to Heaven. Who knows what is right or wrong.

God is good, all the time.

January 26, 2009

As I am crying out to God this morning to not let Steve suffer, I can't help but think about the suffering of Jesus, throughout his life and especially the last three years. Certainly Jesus caught the flu now and then, or drank some tainted water along the road. What about the pebbles in the sandals, splinters from his wood-working and coughing from all of that carpentry dust?

What about the forty days of fasting? I have done fasting, for a day. I think three days was my longest fast. Forty days has to be extremely painful. And on the top of fasting, he was harassed by his worst enemy, taunted, made fun of, emotionally battered. Then His creation, rejected Him, called Him names, spat on Him. He was stripped and whipped, with nails pounded through His hands and feet into pieces of crossed wood, and finally they thrust a spear through his side. He suffered so much, yet all the while His Father watched. All the while His Father felt Jesus' pain and I am sure He wanted it to stop, but it was for a purpose. The suffering had significance. The suffering was for a reason.

I don't know the reason for Steve's suffering. I want it to stop. *Now*. I want a miracle. I want the miracle of healing or the miracle of Heaven. I want Steve to feel good again. It has been a long time since he has really felt good. I am willing, we both are, to do whatever God wants us to do. But this suffering thing is tough. I understand better now how God felt watching His Son physically tormented. It is horrible. If you know the end is in sight, it's so much easier to bear. In twenty-four hours the flu will be over, or next week the antibiotics will have taken care of the Strep Throat. Boy, is it different when there is no end in sight, or knowing as we do that the end could literally be the end of Steve's life and our marriage.

Sometimes God does not show His hand until the bets are made and the hand is over. I don't need to see God's hand. I just want the hand to be over. I want Steve to feel good.

God is good, all the time.

January 27, 2009

I watched my father-in-law, Steve's dad, die. It was just two years ago this month that Tom Sorrelle was diagnosed with Pancreatic Cancer. After considering his options, he opted not to take chemo which would have possibly given him a couple of extra months. Being the incredible man that he was, he gracefully put his life in God's very capable hands, declaring that either God would heal him like He has so many, or God would be opening the door of Heaven. On March 4, 2007, Tom Sorrelle walked through that open door.

I had many questions at the time. Is it better to know when that door will be open, or is it better to go quickly, painlessly, effortlessly, and unknowingly? On the one hand, you get a chance to say goodbye, right all the wrongs, connect one more time with the people you love and the people you haven't seen in a long time, pray, and get your paperwork in order. But a quick death means no suffering, no pain, no agony.

A friend of mine is helping her sister and kids deal with missing their father, who slipped while getting into his hot tub, hitting his head and drowning. In a couple of short, unconscious moments he went from here to there, walking through that open door into a really great place. At just forty-five-years-old, he was too young to die, and his family is shocked and reeling from that moment. He, of course, is happy, really, really happy, but his family misses his presence so much. For him it was easy; here one moment, in paradise the next. It's even better than taking a jet to Cancun from subzero temperatures, ice and snow.

Tom, on the other hand, said his goodbyes, told people he loved them, made sure his wife knew what a treasure she was to him, taught his kids (his other treasures) a few last life lessons, and made sure that everyone he talked to knew how much he loved God. But there was the pain, nausea and suffering.

Sometimes (okay, *all* of the time), God really knows what He is talking about. His wisdom throughout the Bible is unbelievable and hits me when I am not even asking for it. So we are supposed to live every day like there won't be a tomorrow, but what does that mean?

If tomorrow does not come here and I have not made right a relationship or really showed Jesus to everyone with whom I come in contact, then what good is today? If the last conversation I have with a friend is about what someone was wearing or how nasty someone's breathe was, and that's what my friend remembers, what did today mean? Or worse, I condemned someone for who they are and made an enemy because of it, what good am I?

Apparently we don't get to choose. We don't get to pick the quick walk or the slow one, the fast exit or the agonizing one. But we do get to pick how we will make that walk. Causing hurt and pain to people is not what today is about. Today is about hope and healing, living and forgiving, loving and hugging. Today is about tomorrow, which is inevitably about walking through that door to Heaven.

God is good, all the time.

January 31, 2009

Medical Science is not perfect. CAT scans show doctors things they are sure of and others that just create more mystery. So the doctors guess. Sometimes they're right, sometimes they're wrong. Somehow they state their guesses as truth. Then the next doctor comes along with his or her version of "truth." Really, when it comes down to it, a doctor's diagnosis is a reflection of truth—mine can be different than yours, but we can both be honest.

The CAT scan which caused me to be admitted into the hospital this past Tuesday showed an abscess on or near my appendix, which caused my appendix to rupture. Or, the CAT scan showed an abscess that pulled down part of my small bowel and irritated it. Possibly, the scan showed a cavity left over from my hysterectomy, and may contain infection and part of some organ or another.

Either way, I got a four-day, three-night, all-expense paid trip to Butterworth Hospital. The I.V. antibiotics helped lower my white cell count in my blood. Now, at home with more antibiotics, I have a few all-new doctor appointments for next week. I just think that my kidneys had their own version of "Infection Gone Wild" and the kinder, gentler antibiotic did not stop my kidneys attempt at wild partying. Home is great, and my bed at home is even better.

Meanwhile, the love of my life got his first experience at the chemo clinic on Wednesday. (I need to take a moment to say praise God for sisters and sisters-in-law!) The I.V. chemo went pretty well. The pill form, however, was not as agreeable. Steve did not notice the big "TAKE WITH FOOD" alert on the side of the bottle and became nauseated after taking his evening dose. Since discovering and complying with the alert, he feels much better. He's tired, but I think sleep is welcome to him right now.

Today my friend Elena came to clean my house while I take it easy and get better for Steve. She had not seen Steve for a couple of weeks and did not know his diagnosis. Elena asked me why he was yellow (really she said he looked Jell-O in her really cute Spanish accent. I hadn't noticed his yellow tint. To me, Steve still looks like that man standing down at the end of the aisle almost twenty nine years ago, that skinny, string bean of a guy (as my dad called him) in his black tux with the gray striped ascot tie. Never was there a more handsome man in the world. That is my truth, honestly.

God is good, all the time.

February 5, 2009

Yesterday was chemo drip number two. Steve handled it pretty well. During the "input," he had some burning, nausea, yucky feelings, and a bit of wondering if this chemo was doing any good at all.

Afterward we met with Dr. Brinker who reminds us all of a young Groucho Marx, not a bad thing in an oncologist. Dr. Marx (since Dr. Groucho would make him sound like he had an unpleasant disposition, nothing could be further from the truth) had received the second opinion from Dr. Al Benson out of Northwestern University in Chicago. The second opinion highly resembled the first, so onward we go. Steve has six more days of oral chemo followed by a week of no chemo, and then the cycle will repeat. Dr. Marx promised to be completely honest with us. If the chemo is not doing anything, he won't just continue for the sake of giving him more chemo. But, if it is doing some good, then more chemo will be coming.

Steve is currently on seven prescription medications and a couple of over the counter medications, too. It seems that if you take this med you need to take med, and that med will make you (fill in the blank) so now another drug is necessary. I'm in there so often these days they have posted my name under "main dish" for the Walgreens Employee Valentine's Party. Perhaps I should stop wearing a red smock when I go in to pick something up from the pharmacy.

What's happening in our home is so hard. Steve and I have pretty much stopped working, which has led to his feeling useless in the business. The right pills need to be dispensed at the right times. Finding foods that sound good to Steve is a daily challenge. Nausea, vomiting, sleeplessness, restlessness, pain, hiccups, and constipation have taken the place of work, church, socializing, shoveling snow, house repairs, and enjoying regular everyday life. He is still Steve—strong, faithful, loving, and kind. But watching him suffer is the hardest thing I have ever done, and I have done some pretty tough things.

I am trying really hard to live in the day and in the moment. We have had some *really* great moments. It's been a while since we have had a whole good day. But I will take the moments when they come. Today I threatened Steve's bowels. "If you don't move by noon, I am calling the doctor," I warned. That could mean a trip to the hospital or to Walgreen's, but I am hoping that the "Senokot S" and cup of strong coffee will make something move. But bowels or no bowels, his pain is increasing and right now it is impossible to know if it is the chemo or the cancer that are making him feel so crappy.

I have decided I will fight with every ounce of my being to be unselfish. I am not going to be one of those spouses that wants their mate to stay with me so badly I don't let him live. I am not going to make him chase after a cure when none currently exists. I am not going to hang on so tightly to Steve that he can't hear the voice of God when it is time to walk into Heaven.

I will continue to pray for a miracle and be by his side until that miracle happens, trying to make him happy in every way that I can. I will walk beside him as long as he is here with me, making him malts and running to whatever restaurant or grocery store he wants at any moment of the day or night. After all, he was a trooper through four pregnancies, various surgeries, a few kidney stones, and years of PMS. He ran to Meijer for ice cream and pickles, pain killers and tampons. He worked with me, coached by my side and rubbed my back during labor. We are a team. A team sticks together through wins and losses, highs and lows. This team is strong and unbeatable. We have a great coach and He will take us all the way to the championship!

God is good, all the time.

February 8, 2009

In the Gospel of John, there is an account of Mary Magdalene discovering Jesus' empty tomb three days after his crucifixion. She ran to find a couple of His buddies, and when they came back to the cave they discovered that the cloth his body had been wrapped in was crumpled up and tossed to the side. The cloth that had been covering his face, however, was neatly folded and placed on the ground.

In Jewish tradition of that time, a servant would set the master's table and hide away until the master had completely his meal. If the master was finished he would take his napkin, crumple it up and throw it on the table. That was the servant's cue to know it was alright to clear the plates. If he was not yet finished, he would fold the napkin neatly and place it aside. A folded napkin told the servant not to clear the table because the master would be returning.

One little detail in that story makes such a powerful statement. Jesus is not finished; He is coming back. Praise God that during this time of our lives, we know this to be true. Apparently, God is not finished with any one of us yet. Steve is kind of searching for what it is that God still has for him here. Steve's apprehensions are not in dying but in living with this disease. In dying there is victory. When living with pain, it is hard to think about winning.

I do believe God can make amazing things come out of a really crappy situation. I pray that God lets us see some miracles now. I pray everyone who reads this will pray, just for a minute, and really talk to God. I pray you listen to Him after you say your piece. Let Him show you that He is real. Let God wrap His arms around you and hold you while you torment over "why Steve?" or "why me (as in you)?" Let God be the place where you go when the world makes no sense whatsoever. Let Him show you something good that is coming out of all of this junk.

God is good, all the time.

February 10, 2009

One day at a time. That has become my mantra. Today, just today, let there be peace, joy, love, patience and understanding in my home and in my heart.

Today was a good day. The sun was shining and it was a balmy fifty-six degrees outside; no true Michigander would have been caught dead wearing a coat outside. What a great February heat wave! I think I may have even gotten a little bit sunburned.

Today was also the last day that Steve will have chemo for an entire week. I am hoping his chemo-free living will give him back a life. He feels so crummy. Soon we will know if the chemo is the culprit. So, tonight we are looking forward to tomorrow.

Since I am in such a great mood and ready for a party, I decided to plan one. On Saturday, February 28, at 9 a.m., I will be hosting a Painting/Spring Cleaning Party. Anyone who would like to come is welcome. I will provide all of the food and beverages. All of the white trim needs to be touched up and closets, windows, and cupboards need to be cleaned. Steve is thinking that this house is a bit much for us to handle so I am working hard to put it on the market. Please let me know if you plan on coming so that I can plan food, paint brushes, etc. So put on your work clothes and come for a good time.

Here is a word from my son, Noah, a former Navy man working in damage control now in the Army National Guard in the Reserved Officer Training Program. It's amazing how many people ignore the possibility of cancer until someone they know is affected by it. There are many preventative actions that people can take that they normally wouldn't think of hadn't it been for cancer affecting someone they know. Here's Noah's "word": "In 2007, I had a U.S. Navy safety brief before the holiday season. A man came to speak to us with an incredible story. He had been working for an oil company, and his job was to inspect pipelines for leaks. He worked the night shift, and after working there for many years, he became lax on following the rules. One night, he drove his truck to inspect a portion of a pipeline. The rules stated that any vehicles in the vicinity must be turned off during inspection, but he had left it on many times before without an issue. That night, a pipe sprung a terrible leak. The first thing he thought of as oil was spraying him was that he had left his truck on. He ran for his truck, but it had caught on fire before he could reach it. He too burst into flames.

Emergency help arrived, and he was rushed to a burn victim clinic. There, he spent months in agonizing pain. He repeatedly asked himself, "For what?" For what possible reason had this terrible thing happened? And he was right; for *what*? It was an avoidable situation, had he taken the precautions. His story, however, undoubtedly spared many other oil workers from accidents as many likely decided to think twice before committing a safety violation.

I'm not saying that cancer is self-inflicted. There are precautions, however, and they can save your life. With the death of my grandfather two years ago, due to pancreatic cancer, combined with my mother's breast cancer and Steve's adenocarcinoma, many people in our family and outside are getting tested for cancer when they normally wouldn't have bothered. They're also changing their diets to help prevent the formation of cancer. If these tragic events hadn't affected my family, who knows how many others may have developed cancer and found out when it was already too late.

I used to think that the pink ribbons and ribbons of every other color representing all kinds of cancers were cute, but what purpose did they serve? I also questioned the Hollywood fundraisers which raised millions of dollars for cancer research while children are starving in our world. I wondered, *for what*? Now I know it is all for a good reason. Because of money being poured into cancer research, many lives have been spared. Those same lives have helped others live, children eat, women give birth to healthy babies and much more. Many of those people have lived to tell others their story of victory over disease and death.

Whether Steve is here for a couple more months or thirty more years, he plans on living his life in a way that glorifies God. He is living each moment as an adventurous gift, anticipating what wonders today will bring. Steve is looking to the Lord for new lessons and a deeper friendship with Him, not questioning "Why me God?" but instead asking "What now Lord?" Me too—I am asking "What now?"

God is good, all the time.

February 12, 2009

I got up this morning to find that almost all the snow has melted away. Any day in February without snow is a good day.

Steve asked me a question a couple of days ago that has me struggling. "If you were in my position, what would you do?" he said.

Part of me wanted to tell him that I am in his position, we all are. We will all leave this body behind, we just don't know when. But I realized that was a flippant answer. Of course we will all go sometime, but most of us plan on living well into our eighties or nineties.

My next response was that I would go with dignity and grace, floating away peacefully into the arms of Jesus. Nice thought but really hard to do. I watch him living with all of this pain, having difficulty swallowing, days that drag on and on, sleepless nights and battling the body just to do anything, all the while not knowing how much worse things will get or when it will end.

Dignity and grace would be difficult for me. With Steve they seem to be second nature. Really, they are his nature. Steve has always exemplified dignity. He never swears, never has a bad thing to say about anyone. He is honest, faithful, trustworthy and kind. Steve is grace-full in every way. He always shows mercy to those he fathers, works with, and those whom he calls friend. I believe that anyone who knows Steve would be hard pressed to come up with something negative to say about him. Thanks to the hand of God and the work of his parents, Steve is an exceptional man.

More realistically, if I were in Steve's position, I think I would beg God for a miracle. I would attend every healing service and class on miracles that I could find. I would call Benny Hinn and Reinhard Bonnke and ask for a special anointing. I would print up posters with Bible verses that refer to God's healing powers. I would make deals with God, along the lines of this: *I will give the rest of my life in service to Haiti or Burkina Faso, sell my house and live in a hut working with the poor until I was too old to work anymore, if only you make me well.* Or I would promise never to gossip again, to diligently recycle, stop exaggerating the truth and live with my real hair color. All of those promises would certainly lead God to take all of the cancer away.

How do I answer that question? What would *you* do if you were told that the rest of your life is now measured in months?

I want to say let's go to Disney World, eat hot fudge sundaes and candied apples. Let's visit the Dominican Republic and Burkina Faso one last time. Let's go to Paris and Rome and London and other places that we have never been before. Let's sit at a small Parisian café and have lattes and pastries. Let's spend as much time as we can with our kids and grandbabies. Let's go dancing and enjoy everything that this world has to offer. Let's live while we are still together.

That's what Steve is doing. He is living. He does not feel well enough to travel or strong enough to be with people all of the time. He can't eat much or drink much. He is praying for healing but he's not making any deals with God. His faith is full. He is living in the same way he has since I met him thirty years ago. He is a picture of dignity and grace. He is dancing.

God is good, all the time.

February 13, 2009

Happy Valentine's Day Eve! Today the drug store was full of last minute Valentine shoppers buying chocolates and cards. I am proud to say that I finished my shopping nearly a week ago, which is like six weeks in Christmas shopping time.

Dr. Wise paid us a visit today. Things seem to be progressing rather quickly with Steve. I believe it is God's mercy. Days go by so slowly for Steve. Even though it has only been four weeks since this medical nightmare began, I have a hard time remembering life without it.

Besides writing new prescriptions and changing some old ones, Dr. Wise gave us some great advice: "Don't let the cancer define you," he said, "because the cancer is not you." It was a pretty deep thought for a couple of people living on little sleep. Steve is not his cancer, nor is he his symptoms. Steve is a great guy trapped in a crappy body.

I rolled over in bed last night without realizing how close I was to Steve. I made contact with Steve's side. Just lightly, not like a punch or a strong elbow, but just a touch. Steve groaned. This morning he groaned more, not just groaned but also complained, strongly. This morning was the first grumpy moment Steve has had. It is the first time that he complained about anything having to do with his cancer. As part of my oh-so-generous heart, I told him that he could be grumpy today, but just today. After all, tomorrow is Valentine's Day, and no one is allowed to be grumpy on February 14. It is the day we celebrate love and everyone has someone they love. So no grumpy allowed.

Laying down the law was useless. Steve's grumpy only lasted about twenty minutes, tops. I can count on one hand the number of times that Steve has raised his voice at me in all of the years that I have known him. And, quite frankly, I earned every one of them. I have given him plenty of reason to yell, but he usually decided not to. Steve has always taken God's side in any battle. He has always shown me love when I did not deserve it, patience when I pushed him, kindness when I wasn't kind, and Jesus no matter what. Steve makes me a better person.

Steve is a great husband because of his faith in God. God does really wonderful things with people that trust and believe in Him. I happen to be the lucky recipient of lots of those wonderful things.

God is good, all the time.

February 15, 2009

According to my dictionary, the definition of mercy is an act of kindness, compassion or favor or something that gives evidence of a divine favor; a blessing. Mercy is what we are praying for, divine mercy. Mercy is our plea and mercy is what we are receiving.

Valentine's Day was wonderful. Ritalin gave Steve some much missed energy. Steve (with a little help from a certain unnamed sister-in-law) gave me a beautiful heart charm for my favorite bracelet. I gave Steve (again with some help from LeeAnne) his favorite chocolate candy, sea foam. Hallmark did a beautiful job expressing our hearts in cards. Noah and Susie came in for the weekend. Our Amber Jean the Beauty Queen came into town with her Marine husband, whom I adore almost as much as Amber. Cousins Mary and Cheri also visited. Laci came over with my new grand-puppy, Byron, who was the hit of the day, and he hardly even peed on the carpet. Taylor made some of the best French Onion Soup I have ever tasted.

Later in the evening, our good friends Fred and Mary Ellen came over and kicked back, chatting with us about a whole lot of nothing for a good couple of hours. All in all, it was one of the best Valentine's Days we have ever celebrated. That's the good news.

The bad news is that shortly before midnight, our day fell apart. Steve was up all night vomiting. Nothing was bringing relief. I phoned Dr. Wise at 7:30 a.m. and by noon Steve was hooked up to sub-q meds for pain and nausea. I praise God for Dr. Wise. The other good news is he has not thrown up since, and his pain is much better.

Today was a tough day. It started early and is not over yet. But today I learned a lot about bravery. That was today's gift. Perhaps I will share what I learned sometime in the near future. Two of my all-time favorite songs are about mercy: "Mercy Came Running" and "Mercy Seat." Both songs have lyrics which speak of the wonderful, healing mercy of God, free and complete. This is not the first time I have prayed for mercy and, surely, it will not be the last. Right now, however, I need mercy more than I've ever needed it. My prayer is that God shows Steve incredible mercy.

I was sitting on the couch today with Steve praying. As I was begging for mercy, God gently reminded me that He was not waiting for Steve in Heaven, or far away contemplating whether or not to give Steve a miraculous healing. He was there. God was right there on the couch with us, holding us, crying with us, loving us, right there, where we were, and He's also *here*, where you and I are, right now. God is here. God is mercy.

God is good, all the time.

February 16, 2009

I hate roller coasters. I would never go parachuting or bungee jumping. I prefer wild animals in cages to those running loose around me, including all types of snakes, spiders and rodents. I don't want to swim with the sharks. My water skiing days are behind me. Jumping big waves on Lake Michigan makes me nauseous. I don't mind being on the top floor of the Sears Tower; I just can't look out the windows. I would rather blow up balloons than ride in one. I will never watch a scary movie or read a scary book if I am home alone. I shake at the sound of the dentist's drill or the sight of stirrups at the gynecologists. I am a major chicken. Yet, Steve calls me brave.

Today has been better than yesterday. The sunshine helps. The meds are doing their jobs. Not a lot of sleep last night but maybe tonight sleep will come.

Heroes come in all shapes and sizes: the sweet boy that helps his elderly neighbor get her cat out of the tree, a firefighter fighting the flames to save a child's life, a lifeguard, policeman, paramedic, doctor. Heroes bravely sacrifice themselves for the lives of others.

My hero is about six foot three, tall, dark and handsome. He has given his life for me and our kids. My hero diligently seeks to be in the will of God. He has taught me about love, life, fixing toilets and eternity. He has been a stellar example of a man to his sons and has demonstrated what to look for in a husband to his daughter. He stares into the face of adversity and calmly speaks the name of Jesus, his comfort, his strength, his rock. He is the bravest man I have ever known. *My hero.*

Yesterday Steve told me that I was brave, something I have never been accused of before. When I have traveled to places like Haiti and Kenya, I have been told that I am ignorantly trusting, not brave. But maybe facing this double-cancer thing head on is bravery. Perhaps not letting Steve's cancer play a part in our relationship takes courage. I don't know if I am brave, but I do know that I would give up my life for Steve. I want to be Steve's hero.

God is good, all the time.

February 18, 2009

February 18 is another decision day. After hours of prayer and great medical advice from Dr. Wise and Dr. Marx, Steve is switching to full hospice care. Dr. Marx advised against another round of chemo, at least at this time. The last round really put Steve into a tail spin he is having a hard time coming out of. Sometimes chemo helps, sometimes it hurts. If Steve starts feeling better in a few weeks, he can always sign up for another round.

I used to hear the word "hospice" and cringe. Hospice is that service you get when all hope is gone, and death is knocking at the door. Now I realize that hospice can bring hope. Maybe not *bring* hope, but allow hope. With chemo the hope is that modern medicine can take care of the disease. With hospice, only God can make the disease go away. Let go and let God. That is where we are right now, letting go of medical hope and letting God work a miracle.

I am so looking forward to what God has in store for us. The idea of a miracle that will wipe away all the cancer is so thrilling and exciting. To think that one day, in the not-so-distant future, Steve will be dancing like he used to (disco was his genre), teaching kids how to play volleyball and golf, going out on a tractor to make sure that the greens are cut just so, setting up tables for a big banquet, playing "play run" with the grandbabies, and beating whoever he plays at tennis. What a picture. What joy!

I have no doubt that Steve will be healed of this cancer. I just don't know if his healing will happen here and give me forty more years of being his dance partner, or if I will have to wait until we are both in heaven to try out our dance steps again. Either way, the miracle will happen. Either way, I will be with Steve. Either way, God gets the glory.

God is good, all the time.

February 20, 2009

Some of my very favorite stores are Barnes and Noble, Schuler's Books and Music, and Family Christian Book Store. I have spent hours perusing the shelves, looking at book after book, trying to decide what to buy. If I am going somewhere I have never been before, I buy a travel book. If there is a subject I want to know more about, I buy the book. If one of my favorite authors comes out with a new novel, I buy the book. If there is a new, easy way to lose weight, I buy the book.

But even with all the time I have spent going up and down the aisles, there is a book I have not found. I really need a book on how to do *this*. I want a step-by-step, day-by-day guide on how to deal with all of the different emotions and moods associated with facing a terminal illness. I need to find out exactly how to make Steve happy, how much laughter is appropriate and when it is alright to cry. I would like there to be a chapter on how to get by on very little sleep, and another one on how to cook meals that taste great but omit no cooking smells. The book also needs to have a list of go-to conversation topics that do not create added anxiety. Some medical terms would also be useful as would directions on dealing with sub-q medications, button needle sights and the best prescriptions on the market. It would be great to have a list of responses to give to people who think they know the way to cure cancer, obtain marijuana without a prescription and what spiritual healer is currently getting the biggest results.

A portion of the book should focus on when it is alright to be human and when superhuman strengths are needed. Included should be a how-to section on sponge baths, foot massages and pillow positioning. I am sure there is more I would want in the book, but right now I am too tired to think of what that is.

Steve is doing really well today. Last night was the best night's sleep that either of us has had in a long time. An afternoon nap helped perk Steve up even more. Days like this seem pretty normal after some of the rotten days he has had. Somehow it is easier to feel God when things are going better.

Hospice came today to sign Steve up to the program. They do have a lot to offer. Although hospice is wonderful and will be a huge support, I am looking forward to the day we can tell them we don't need them anymore because the cancer is gone. I am looking forward to that celebration.

My hat's off to the West Catholic Girls Varsity Basketball Team, who not only beat their opponent last night but in doing so raised lots of money for Gilda's Club. Thanks so much to Sami and the rest of the team for giving breast cancer another kick in the pants. Thanks so much for including me in your great night. If you guys need me to give you an extra tough practice or inspiring pep talk before districts, give me a call. I will come running! Thanks, too, for letting me forget about "real life" for a few hours. You guys played great, and you are a classy team on and off the floor.

God is good, all the time.

February 22, 2009

Today started at 4 a.m. The sound of the side door opening woke me from a pretty good sleep. Steve had decided that the cars needed to be repositioned in the driveway. He did that before I even got out of bed. Since West Michigan was blessed with several inches of snow on Saturday, Steve also wanted to shovel for a while but the combination of the cold and my nagging brought him inside.

There are times when I look into Steve's eyes and I see someone else. I don't know who it is, but I do know Steve is not there. Those times are becoming more frequent. Whoever it is in Steve's body sounds just like Steve, but does not act the way he would or say the things that he would say. The voice pretends to know me, but the tongue is much sharper than Steve's. I don't know where Steve goes when the voice takes over, but I hope it is someplace warm and sunny, joyful and free of illness, a happy place like Disney World or an all-inclusive resort in the Dominican Republic.

As I look for the joy of today, the little miracles along the way, I think that this is one of them. Steve's little vacations help him to get through the long days. I wish that I could go with him. I would love to lose myself in the wonder of the Magic Kingdom or forget about everything while sipping something cool with sand under my feet. Steve and I have taken some great vacations over the years. I am really glad we didn't put that off until our retirement.

God truly is good. Last week Steve prayed that someone would come over and help. Soon after, his brother came over and fixed a few things. Just when I start to feel down, the phone rings and a friendly voice lets me know that I am not alone. God seems to help me open a book to the right place or the Bible to the right passage which brings comfort and renewed hope. Our "Joy Jar" always has something important for each day. Any time I need a reminder that God is here, He gently taps me on the shoulder and lets me fall into His arms.

God is good, all the time.

February 24, 2009

Four days until the most fun Painting and Cleaning Party ever (I hope)! I am still planning on 9 a.m. or whatever time people can come. I will have my list and supplies ready. I so appreciate the response and willingness to help with the house. Having things spruced up and ready to go will be such a relief. Man, our friends are awesome!

Changing the topic, then, I want to tell you about the time when Amanda was three and she started having seizures. (Now she is twenty six, but I am only twenty nine, so I am not sure how I could have a daughter who is twenty six. You know, fifty is the new thirty, so I will be turning thirty about the same time she does.)

Anyway, her seizures were violent and deeply affected her life. As we took her from one doctor to the next, from University of Michigan to Cleveland Clinic to Mayo Clinic, Amanda always told everyone she met that Jesus was going to heal her. Amanda never doubted, never questioned, never complained. When she talked about her expected miracle, there was joy and excitement in her voice. Knowing that Jesus loved her, she knew He would not let her down. Jesus came through for her when she was eight years old. No more seizures, EEGs, medicine, blood tests or doctors. The miracle, the one that she had anticipated for five long years, was finally hers.

Yesterday several 5th and 6th grade students from Tri-Unity Christian School visited us to pray for us. That's the school my children attended and where we coached for years. They were young kids with young hearts full of faith. A few of them brought verses to share to which God had directed them. One young man, River, shared how Jesus told people that if they have faith, incredible things can happen. "Jesus said that if you have faith and tell a mountain to move, it will move." River pointed out that mountains might not be just physical mountains but can be other obstacles in our lives like cancer. Then they prayed, believing that Jesus will move that cancer mountain. The prayer was every great emotion wrapped up together like the most beautiful present you have ever received. It was not just a pretty package, but an awesome gift with perfect timing and orchestration.

When Steve's dad was walking this same road with this same cancer two years ago, his faith was amazing. I asked Steve then how his dad could be so peaceful. He reminded me that Jesus said that He is the "author and finisher of our faith." That verse never meant much to me until that time. Jesus was bridging the gap. He was standing in between life here and Heaven, bridging the fear of death and the unknown. That middle part, the fear part, was no longer part of Tom. His faith was complete.

Like Amanda's story teaches me, the faith of a child is complete, no cynics or critics or cruelties of life have interfered with their belief yet.

After Steve was diagnosed we prayed for a word from God. Finally the word came, complete. One word, full of meaning: Steve is complete.

Jesus, you complete me.

God is good, all the time.

February 25, 2009

The last couple of days have been great. Steve is stronger than he has been since before going into the hospital in January. He is sleeping better, eating more and getting his focus back. He even watched a little bit of the Military Channel on T.V. yesterday. We might even watch a movie if there's a good one on.

I've been thinking lately about birthdays. When I was a kid, my birthday was the best day of the year. I would start to think about it a couple of months ahead of time. I would daydream about birthday cake, a special gift and getting five dollars in the mail from Grandma Fouty. My parents always made our birthdays special. The whole family would go to Meijer Thrifty Acres on Alpine Avenue. My brothers and I would go to the upper level cafeteria for a red pop while my parents shopped in the toy section, the best section, of the store. Bruce, Joel and I would hang over the railing, craning our necks to see if we could steal a peek at what Mom and Dad were putting in their cart. I don't remember ever spotting them but we got a lot of exercise trying.

There was one year that I asked for a dancing ballerina doll. My parents were great at getting us what we asked for, so I had a spot in my bedroom ready for that doll's arrival. Sitting at the dining room table with my birthday cake as the centerpiece, I grew more anxious for that beautiful doll in the pretty pink tutu. As I opened the customary preliminary small gifts, a pot-holder loom, brownie refills for my Easy Bake Oven, Barbie's latest groovy outfit, anticipation zoomed. But where was the doll? Suddenly, my parents "remembered" that there was one last gift hidden on the basement stairs. Here it was, the box holding the beautiful crowned dancer, wrapped in Looney Tunes wrapping paper. I carefully opened each end, wanting the moment to last forever. Tearing the tape ever so carefully, I saw the picture on the side of the box. What was this? As I tore of the last piece of paper, reality hit. This was not my doll, the only thing I truly wanted for my tenth birthday. This was the all-important birthday that brought me into double digits. The birthday, unlike any others, that took me from little girl to young lady. I spent my whole summer dreaming of this doll, to me a treasure. September is a long time to wait for such an extraordinary gift. But I didn't un-wrap a doll; instead, I un-wrapped an orange AM/FM radio. I never asked for a radio. The only songs I knew were the ones my mom played on our 8-Track, the ones sung by Engelbert Humperdinck, Tom Jones and The Temptations. That music was clearly "mom" music. I didn't have any music. What was I going to do with a radio?

Soon that question was answered when my mom told me that I was too old for dolls and the radio would last me a long time. Pasting a fake smile on my face, I took the knife out of my heart and put the batteries into the radio. That day I started listening to WGRD, memorizing lyrics, and groovin' to the beat. September 3, 1971, was the beginning of my musical journey in life. I began listening to the Eagles, Chicago, Billy Joel, Elton John, Michael Jackson, The Carpenters, Boston, Journey, Styx, Melissa Manchester, Sonny and Cher, Simon and Garfunkel, Crosby, Stills and Nash, and many more artists I still enjoy today. That orange radio was turned on every morning while I got ready for school and every evening when I went to my room for the night. From 5th grade until I got married, that radio was a constant friend through cute boys and heartaches, happy times and sad, victories and defeats.

Somehow my mom and dad knew what I had asked for, the ballerina doll, was not really what was best for me. Somehow God knows, too. He knows that what we ask for is not necessarily the best thing for us. But in the end, He gives us what is best.

God is good, all the time.

February 26, 2009

Steve is back! The wonderful man that I married has returned to me, fully. It's as if the disease does not exist. Just a couple of days ago, I really thought that everything was happening so fast and I would not have Steve to kiss and hold for very long. Today I feel like we will have the next thirty years together.

Target and Meijer were both graced with Steve's presence this morning as we had our first outing in a long time. We bought compression socks for swollen feet, some small surprises for our grandbabies' "treasure boxes" and mouse traps.

I have a theory about the mice. I think that they heard that our kids all moved out and figure we now have room for them. Mice should live outside. Hopefully they will see the traps and make a beeline for the door.

On our trip, Steve wore his St. Patrick's Day Snoopy pajama pants, a striped polo shirt and some tennis shoes. After a sweet woman walked by and greeted him as if he were a young boy, I realized that we probably looked like a man and a caretaker from an adult foster care facility. I know that because last Christmas we gave similar PJ bottoms and shirts to bless some adult foster care guys through Hope Network. It's funny how we no longer care about what we wear, although I will pick out his clothes from now on.

Since Steve has been so coherent the last couple of days, we have been able to have some great conversations. Most of our talk has centered on his life and how he wants to live it.

Today is the first time Steve cried since his diagnosis, but not for the reasons that someone might think. Steve cried because he is so humbled by God answering so many prayers, humbled by friends being so giving of their time and humbled by family giving so freely of their love. We both are.

Steve's main concern is about other people. He wants to know that his life has not inhibited anyone from knowing God. He needs people to know that he is deeply sorry for harming anyone in any way. He seeks forgiveness for any wrongdoings or shortcomings. Steve's desire, above all else, is that God be glorified through his life, be it short or long. Steve is on his face before the Lord each day, begging to be in the center of His will, to know that each step, each word is right in sync with God's plan. Steve wants so badly to share with everyone his faith in God, the very center point of his life.

"Do you think more people will come to know God through my living or my dying?" Steve asked me today. I don't know the answer, but I do know Steve is willing to do whichever so that more people can know God's saving grace. I also know that if anyone wonders how to know God like Steve does, it's really simple. Just recognize that God exists, He created and loves you and His son, Jesus, is God made man to die on the cross, fulfilling so many scriptures. He then rose from the grave to redeem each one of us who believes. That's it. Believe. Then with belief comes a desire to live for Him. It's really simple, but it does take faith, believing in something you have not seen. That being said, if you have seen Steve, you have seen a glimpse of Jesus. Jesus and Steve are pretty tight.

God is good, all the time.

February 28, 2009

There is something very special about a room full of one gender. Fill a room with a group of women and the conversation begins. The common threads that bind my gender together allows for conversation to flow seamlessly. Women have no problem talking about kids and grandkids, discussing their passions, tearing up regarding their compassions, and finding commonality in the habits of their partners. You'd be hard pressed to put ten wives in a room together and not find out eight of them have to pick up men's underwear from the bathroom floor every day. Those same ten women would also find the antics of a three year old "absolutely darling" and cry together at the thought of a child that same age not having enough food to eat in Haiti. That's what we do—women bond.

Men, on the other hand, talk sports, slap each other's backs, compare cars and pound their chests like Tarzan. At least that's what I have been told. Men bond, too.

Once you throw men and women together in the same room, everything changes. Topics turn from cute toddler antics to politics, from raising money for world hunger to saving money for a new boat. The kids are still discussed, just without such glowing reports.

Somehow men and women do not bond when they're in a mixed group. To achieve that bond, that special relationship between genders, you have to marry one of them. Then the magic can begin.

I remember the day early in our union when I decided I wanted to have a happy marriage. I had seen many couples together, some happy, some not so much. I wanted *happy*. I knew it was up to me. I knew if I would just give of myself, unselfishly, that Steve and I could have a great relationship. It was that day that I decided I would do everything I could to make Steve happy. I started picking up his favorite candy or ice cream when I would go grocery shopping. I tried my hardest not to nag. I cleaned the house, did the dishes, enjoyed making nice meals and even picked up his dirty underwear without complaint. Or at least I made those things my goals. I decided if I could help to make Steve really happy, our marriage would follow suit. It worked. It really, really worked.

My decision was a big turning point in our marriage; probably one that should have happened much sooner, like when we said "I do." That's when I should have embraced the attitude to really please Steve in every way. Unfortunately, at age eighteen, I was just too selfish. Steve, on the other hand, said "I do" for real. He was never the issue. It took me a while to realize that Steve had always been unselfish, giving himself fully to me, to us. So when I did the same, the magic happened.

I am so happy I made the decision to please Steve. I am so grateful we did not wait until the kids were gone to start enjoying each other. I am so thankful that we took trips, enjoyed weekend overnights, laughed, walked, biked and played tennis together. God made our bond grow stronger. It took a while, but I now understand what Scripture means by "the two shall become one."

God is good, all the time.

March 1, 2009

How can I possibly say "Thank you" with enough emphasis? Yesterday's Painting and Cleaning Party was unbelievable. Literally, I would not have believed it had I not seen it myself. The woodwork is white again, the cupboards look brand new, there is no sign of Aurora's artwork on the wall, the floor is now visible in Steve's tool room, cabinets and closets are cleaned, dresser painted, desk organized and bathrooms spotless. And that was just the first two hours! Everyone worked so hard and the quality of the work was so professional. Steve came home from the cottage and walked through the house, amazed at the transformation. To say that we are overwhelmed would be an understatement. Thank you from the bottom of our hearts!

On a discouraging note, things have started to go a bit downhill for Steve. I have to admit, I'm not very optimistic about Friday's CAT scan results, which we should know by tomorrow. Steve's tumors seem more apparent than ever, not because I could see them but because of how he was behaving.

His feet and legs are quite swollen, his pain is increasing and his mind is starting to drift again, so conversation is tougher.

The good news is, like the Veggie Tales say, "God is bigger than the Boogie Man" (or "Boogity Man" for any Seinfeld fans). "Don't tell God how big the mountain is," my new friend, Sue, said to me, "but rather tell the mountain how big God is." Well, we do have a big mountain, but compared to the power and wonder of God, our mountain is really just a mole hill.

I keep trying to tell God how He works. I have reminded Him that the Bible tells us stories about how He healed the blind, lame, lepers and deaf instantly when they asked for a healing. I want instant healing for Steve, no waiting. But then I'm reminded that, for Paul, the healing did not come that readily. Job suffered. Joseph was thrown in a pit and then in jail before he got a really good job (even though he had a cool coat). It took Noah years to build that Ark; the blisters on his hands must have been huge. Sampson got a haircut and lost a lot more than just hair. And Moses' hair turned gray overnight (my worst nightmare).

Even though the healing has not happened overnight, there is good coming from this suffering. Steve and I are closer than we have ever been. People have touched our lives in bigger ways than we could have ever imagined. God has shown us favor, love, kindness, generosity and much, much more.

It is a privilege to rub Steve's feet, fix anything he wants to eat, and help clean and dress him. It is truly a pleasure to rub lotion on his cracked hands, get his medicine ready at bedtime and make sure that his favorite pajamas are cleaned for the next day. He still is and always will be the love of my life, the light of my days and the comfort of my nights. He is Steve, and I am blessed. I am honored to be called Mrs. Stephen Sorrelle. I love you, Babe.

God is good, all the time.

March 3, 2009

One snowy December afternoon, when my kids were much younger, they were laying down watching Irving Berlin's "White Christmas" while I was making dinner. The next thing I knew Luke, then just three years old, started vomiting. I ran him into the bathroom where he began to convulse. It was not hard to recognize what was happening because I had seen it so many times before with Amanda. Luke was having his first Grand Mal seizure.

I flipped out. As soon as it was safe for him, I laid Luke on the couch, wrapped in a blanket. I ran to my room to change clothes so that I could take him to the Emergency Room. I shut my bedroom door and cursed out Satan. I was so angry that this was happening again, to another one of my babies. I yelled at Satan, told him how much I despised him and how he had no right to have anything to do with my family. I screamed at Satan because my screams needed to be directed at someone, and he was a really easy target.

Since I had already been through all of this with Amanda, I would have expected to react differently. I knew what was happening physically to Luke. I understood what I needed to do next, what doctor to call, what medicines were available and what tests would be needed. I was prepared for this because of what life had already thrown my way.

But this time I was emptied. I could not believe I was getting the same diagnosis for one of my children all over again.

Tonight I am reliving that moment and that feeling of emptiness. Tonight we got the CAT scan results from last Friday. Denial, or maybe just wanting so badly for Steve to be alright, had me hoping beyond hope that his original diagnosis was just a mistake. I have been praying that the doctors were wrong, that the January CAT scan really showed just a shadow. I wanted that miracle; the cancer gone and life beginning again.

The test results show no improvement from the last. The cancer is still there, still ugly, nasty and doing its darnedest to destroy Steve's body.

I feel like we got the same diagnosis all over again. I feel the same kick in the stomach, tears on my face, and the feeling of breath being sucked out of my body. I am *pressed*. But not crushed. Persecuted not abandoned. Struck down but not destroyed. Because I am blessed beyond this disease, beyond pain, beyond hurt. For God's promise is eternal. His joy will be my strength. Though the sorrow may last through the night, His joy comes in the morning. I'm trading my sorrow, shame, sickness and pain for the joy of the Lord. And we say yes Lord. Amen.

God is good, all the time.

March 5, 2009

How do you live life with no regrets? I regret yelling at my kids out of my own frustration rather than their bad behavior, cheating on diets, losing touch with friends that mean so much to me. I regret missing opportunities to help someone and the major and minor sins of my past. I regret not spending enough time outside in the summer when winter is here. I regret not being as God-honoring with my money as I should be. I regret making fun of kids when I was in grade school. I regret blaming my PMS on Steve. I regret wearing leg warmers in the 70's, large shoulder pads in the 80's, whitewashed jeans in the 90's and getting a "tramp stamp" tattoo in 2002. (At least the tattoo washed off with a little soap and water. The other fashion regrets are forever captured on film.)

I wish that I could turn back the hands of time and redo so many days, hours, and moments of my life. I wish I could have some do-over's, some mulligans. *I wish.*

I do believe it is not so much the stupid things we do, but how we act afterward when we recognize we have been stupid. God is more concerned with our reaction to our misdeeds then the misdeeds themselves. Sins are a heart issue and God is all about the heart. He wants to know where our heart is: "Where your heart is, your treasure will be also." Or, as we say these days, "Put your money where your mouth is." If our heart is right, our intensions, passions, loves, desires, and actions will follow.

Guilt isn't just for Catholic penance and Jewish mothers. We all experience guilt. Even though we know we are forgiven, we still feel bad about the action that required forgiveness. That little pit in our stomachs is a great reminder of what not to do again. It's the pit-less people that need to be pitied, those who feel no remorse after hurting others.

Pits can shrink. Time helps to shrink pits. Spending time serving, helping, loving, praying and recognizing the accomplishments of others can shrinks the pit faster. Asking for forgiveness and vowing to not repeat past "pit causers" helps them to go away the quickest.

Steve has regrets, but not very many since he gave his heart to Jesus. He has tried to walk uprightly, love fully, give generously and live unselfishly. I am one blessed woman.

God is good, all the time.

March 6, 2009

The last couple of days have been tough. Steve is slipping back into that non-Steve personality that I don't know very well. Pain is higher so the meds are increased. Sleep is difficult at night and unwelcome during the day.

I used to think that disease was purely physical, so therefore the symptoms of illness were also just that. Now I realize that the physical cannot be separated from the spirit (soul) part of us. Anxiety that goes along with a nasty diagnosis is not merely mental or emotional but also physical and spiritual. The emotional takes a toll on the body no matter how strong our spirit is.

What's interesting is that as Steve's body fades his spirit grows stronger. His longing for the things of heaven is replacing his love for the things of earth. Prayers escape his lips with nearly every exhale. His conversations with God are constant and friendly, like sitting down and having a cup of coffee with a really close friend. Steve insight is deep and powerful. His words, when talking about God and eternity, are full of wisdom. Passages from the Bible have new meaning and words to spring to life from the pages.

It's all starting to make sense. We are physical beings with a spirit. Even though we may focus on one or the other, even ignore one or the other, the fact that we are both physical and spiritual cannot be denied. The question is, do we recognize both?

God is good, all the time.

March 8, 2009

God in His incredible mercy is holding Steve in His abundant arms. Jesus took Steve into His presence this morning. No more pain, no more suffering.

Thank you for your loving kindness shown through prayers and support these last few months. May God richly bless you for all the love you have shown me and my family, and Steve.

God is good, all the time.

March 9, 2009

On the night before last, Steve's health took a turn for the worse. Until then, his I.V. meds had kept him pretty comfortable. But after he woke up from a long nap because of abdominal pain, it was obvious the meds could no longer keep up with the destruction that was going on in his body.

After losing his entire day's food intake in the bowl next to his bed, it took from 9:00 p.m. until about midnight to get Steve comfortable enough to sleep. At 5:00 a.m. I woke up to Steve's labored breathing. His inhales were gasps for air and his exhales were painful moans. After contacting the hospice nurse, I went back in the room just in time to see Steve begin to vomit and fall from the bed. As I held Steve while he was writhing in pain on the floor, Noah and Susie tried to get him cleaned up and comfortable. I prayed and begged for the mercy of God. Shortly after the nurse arrived, Joel and LeeAnne walked through the door. Joel tenderly lifted Steve back onto the bed. With pillows propped up behind us, I held Steve close and prayed with him. I told him it was alright to go, that it was time and Jesus would walk with him the whole way.

During that time, Steve took his last breath here on earth and breathed his first in Heaven. God answered my prayers and my pleas. Mercy came running! I have watched people suffer for so long before they died, I am so grateful that Steve's suffering was so short. Thank you Lord for such mercy! And thank you that your mercies are new every morning.

I can just picture Steve wallowing in the presence of God, bathing in His glory. I love to think about the moment he saw his dad and they embraced. And the moment my mom walked up to him, hugged him and thanked him for being such a great husband to her daughter and father to her grandchildren. Also waiting were grandparents, aunts, uncles, cousins and friends. I like to think about him meeting his brothers and sisters who were taken to Heaven so early due to miscarriages. I am awestruck to think of Steve meeting Moses, Abraham, David, Elijah, Paul and his namesake, the Apostle Stephen. All of these saints entered Heaven before him and are now celebrating alongside him, basking in the glow of our God.

Congratulations Steve, you have truly arrived! Love you and miss you, Babe.

God is good, all the time.

Steve Sorrelle Obituary

On August 14, 1957, Stephen Michael Sorrelle was born to Thomas and Nancy (Crowley). At the age of 16, Steve confessed his faith in God and His Son, our Savior, Jesus. He drew power from his faith and chose a life to honor God. God, in His faithfulness, walked with Steve through to the end of his battle with Adenocarcinoma as Steve took his last breath on Earth, followed immediately by his first breath in Heaven. After fifty one years on Earth, Steve is now enjoying a party with those who have gone before him: his dad, Tom, his mother-in-law, Mary (Langlois), some aunts, uncles and friends.

Although we already miss him, we are excited for his celebration. We love you Steve! Devotedly, your wife, Kim (Langlois) Sorrelle; your kids, Amanda Sorrelle, Paul and Laci Sorrelle (DeWeerd), Luke and Megan Sorrelle (Wisniewski), and Noah and Susie Sorrelle (Mercier-Lefebvre); "Adopted Children" Amber (Wesley) and Matt Downer and Cristian & Sarah Santiago (Black)along with many others that you loved and treated as your own, and your grandchildren, Crichton, Aurora, Evayah, Cordelia & Leo, and your Mom and Dad, Thomas Sorrelle who is dancing with you now, and Nancy (Crowley) Sorrelle.

Also remembering Steve are Kim's parents, Bruce and Joanne Langlois and Mary Langlois who went to Heaven before you, your brothers, sisters, nieces, nephews; Michelle, Jenny and Dean Jennings; Robert, Valerie (Rhodes) and Cameron Sorrelle; Renee, Bob and Erin Batt; Patrick, Amanda (Gravelyn), Harrison, Marguerite and Gillian Sorrelle; Andrea, Reese, Mia and Christian (Sorrelle) VanHeck; Jennifer, Tom and Guinevere

Overly; Aimee and Melvin Church; Darryl and Lynda Symanski. Kim's brothers, sisters, nieces, nephews: Joel and LeeAnne (Steil) Langlois, Tessa, Carter, Lindsey, Taylor and Aaron; Bruce and Stacy (VanAllsburg) Langlois, Bruce, Brian, Kelsey and Marc, and the many friends and family members whose lives have changed by knowing you.

March 12, 2009

What a celebration! The last three days have been a great reunion of people who knew and loved Steve. On Monday, many people got together to create a video of memories. We talked and laughed for hours. On Tuesday, hundreds of us gathered at English Hills to share stories, apologize for losses, and remember all of the great things about Steve. Then Wednesday, Pastor Tim and Pastor Sam set the tone to truly celebrate not only Steve's life but his incredible entry into Heaven. Mary and Amber sounded like angels lifting their voices to God in praise and to Steve in appreciation for a life well served. As the video was shown, it was so obvious how much Steve was loved and respected for his service to the Lord, thus service to others. God choreographed a beautiful dance by Cheri and Brie that I believe was mimicked by angelic dancers while Steve watched with his dad, my mom and Aunt Maggie.

We did it. We celebrated. We laughed and cried, and we prayed and praised, all for you, Babe.

Several times the Bible says that "The two shall become one" and even "the two shall become one flesh." Part of me has been ripped away. But God's grace is filling the void, the empty space that was filled by Steve just a couple of days ago. God knows exactly how much grace I need today and He is faithful to deliver.

I miss Steve so much. I miss his smile. I miss beautiful eyes. I even miss his corny jokes and morning breath. I miss seeing his socks on the floor, his toothpaste on the bathroom sink and his cereal bowl in the sink. Above all, I miss the closeness. Cuddling on the couch watching T.V., spooning in bed, holding hands, praying together, kisses on my forehead. I miss the touch.

But my overwhelming feeling right now is complete joy for Steve. I am so happy for him that I am nearly jealous. To be free, completely free, from the junk and bondages of this world and to be in the presence of God is to truly be alive, fully conscious, fully aware, fully living. Go you, Steve. You did it right, running the race and keeping your eye on the goal, and now your reward is eternal joy. Congratulations, Baby!

God is good, all the time.

March 15, 2009

I have spent the last week in a cocoon, shielded from the pain of Steve's leaving. Slowly, the cocoon is now unwrapping, exposing me to the world as it is now, a place without my beloved.

Although I still feel somewhat protected, headaches are becoming more frequent, my nerves are a bit more frayed and my short term memory is nearly nonexistent, as reality is beginning to consume me. One of the hardest things for me to fathom is "life goes on."

I remember being in Meijer shortly after my mom died. As I was absentmindedly filling my cart, I looked around at other people who were doing the same. The difference was they were completely oblivious to my pain. They smiled, chatted, and sped along the aisles without a care in the world, while I had a hard time choosing even the simplest staples for my family's meals. I wondered how this could be. How could they be so light and cheery when I was so weighed down by sorrow and mourning? I remember looking at a gallon of milk. The date was October 3, 14 days after my mom died. I wondered if life would be any better by the time the milk expired. I prayed that it would. That day I left my cart in an aisle and ran to my car. I couldn't do it. I just could not stay in that store. The pressure of the crowd and their oblivion, and the choices that needed to be made about milk and eggs and such were too much.

I have tried since that time to be more sensitive to people in the grocery store. Since no one wears a widow's veil or mourning clothes anymore, we really don't know who is suffering. What a blessing and a burden it would be to know exactly who to reach out to when.

As I was praying this morning, something that Steve and I had promised each other a bit ago came to mind: Take it one day at a time. That's what I have to do now. I need to live for today, pray for today, laugh, love, take a couple of Tylenols and make it through.

My greatest comfort comes from picturing Steve in Heaven.

The last couple of weeks Steve and I talked a lot about Heaven. Steve's theory is that time and the concept of time are totally different there. He is sure that even though I may live another thirty or forty years, to Steve it will be like I walked into the gates right after him. I like that idea. Maybe he will be somewhat familiar with the lay of the land so that he can give me a tour. But I like the idea of following Steve in and spending the rest of our lives together.

So, right now life is happening one day at a time. Pretty soon I hope to graduate to one milk expiration date at a time. The milk in the refrigerator is dated March 23. I think I can make it.

God is good, all the time.

March 19, 2009

I got a few hours of sleep last night. After visiting my primary care physician yesterday, stocking up on prescriptions for sleep, stress, and a sinus infection, I actually slept for about six uninterrupted hours. I attribute the sleep to either the medicines or the great "Dominican Cures Everything Tea" made by Sarah. Either way, it was a great night.

The doctor's appointment yesterday was very interesting. She told me that people often experience panic attacks, false heart attacks, staying in bed for a few days at a time, stress over kids, money, bills, jobs and life in general when their spouse goes to Heaven before them. My doctor said these are not signs that someone is going crazy, just that the body is over-making adrenaline for a while and needs to get back to normal.

I haven't had any of those symptoms yet, so I am still not crazy and will not be crazy if I get the symptoms, which is good because from what I hear crazy is not so great. Plus, I think my kids would let me know if I was going crazy. Or maybe I am crazy, and because I am crazy, I don't know it. So far, no men in white coats have come knocking. I hope that they don't because I don't think that white is my color, plus I know that the sleeves would be way too long on the jacket, even if they buckle them behind my back.

My inner conflict remains the same: I am so happy for Steve, yet miss him so much. It is like mixing Brussels sprouts with cotton candy, or putting snow on a Caribbean beach. Or winning second place in a state championship, at first you are so happy just to have made it into the finals, but when the final buzzer sounds, causing the other team to celebrate ecstatically, all of the air is sucked out of your lungs and complete devastation sets in.

Right now I am just trying to be so happy for the winner, the champion, Steve. He is holding on to the Big Trophy, sitting in the winner's circle. The celebration for Steve is better than any party I have ever thrown, including his fiftieth birthday party, which was a really good one, if I do say so myself. I am so happy for you Babe. I miss you.

God is good, all the time.

March 20, 2009

I have really tried to like camping. I have gone so far as to purchase a tent, sleeping bag, air mattress, special camping pillow, lantern, bug spray, battery powered reading light and a book on "comfort camping" (yeah, right). By the time I paid for everything, I realized the tent is the cheap part. The other stuff can kill a checking account.

I once spent a night in a tent with my cousins in my grandparent's back yard. I learned a lot in that one night: tents do not come with attached bathrooms, every time a tent is unzipped bugs come in, there are sounds outside that I have never heard inside a house, even neighborhoods have bears and coyotes and that an air mattress does not make the ground level.

On the other hand, I can very comfortably spend a few nights in a luxury R.V. in a great campground with a heated pool, health spa and restaurant. I have been told, however, that a classy home on wheels does not count as camping.

This morning my great friend, Sheila, reminded of a Bible verse that was quoted at Steve's service. "For we know that when this earthly tent we live in is taken down—when we die and leave these bodies—we will have a home in heaven, an eternal body made for us by God himself and not by human hands" (2 Corinthians 5:1 NLT).

Paul refers to our bodies as tents. In camping the tent holds us, protects us from some rain and gives us a false sense of security. The tent holds us, the real us. We are not the tent; the tent is just our temporary shelter. Tents get holes and would have a very hard time protecting us from a tornado or hurricane or the Chainsaw Massacre-ist.

Steve's tent did not survive the monsoon. But Steve did. He is in Heaven. For this I am eternally grateful.

I am so happy to know that this body is temporary. Besides the normal physical failings of getting older like wrinkles, extra moles, joint aches and gray hair, I have some other physical failings brought on by my life style. Stretch marks, fat from too much food, sun damage, metal in my teeth due to "Big Daddy Bubble Gum" (watermelon flavor, of course), among other unspeakable abuses, have turned the perfect, soft-skinned body I had as a baby into a body that looks okay in clothing but needs the lights off when undressing.

I am looking forward to a new body in Heaven. I hope that it is five foot six, size four with long brown hair and green eyes.

But I am not ready for that just yet. I have too many things to do here before I can go there. I guess I will just have to change in the dark for a while.

God is good, all the time.

March 24, 2009

I was a couple. My life was the life of a couple. For nearly thirty years (including almost a year of engagement before saying the vows) I have been a couple. When I want to do something, go somewhere, pick out a movie, I check with Steve. I know that Steve would rather have a deluxe pizza than Chinese. I couldn't bribe him into going to a fondue restaurant, but a steak house is a different story. I power shop rather than browse because Steve is either waiting outside the dressing room or at home hoping I will be there soon. I don't order my own ice cream; instead, I just have a few bites of Steve's banana split. No matter where we are, I sleep on the left side of the bed, and he sleeps on the right. He takes out the trash, gets the sprinkler system going in the spring, changes the bags on the vacuum cleaner and knows which rattle means what on the cars. I do the dishes, sweep the floor, pay the bills and pick up his dirty socks and boxers.

I am single. I hate to even say the word. I don't know what single is. I was eighteen when I got married, and before that I was joined at the hip with Sheila and was way too busy to understand single. I still think I need to check in with Steve if I am out and about. I don't know what kind of movies I like, except I thought I liked super hero movies, but it turns out they are really not my thing.

I think that I would rather have Chinese or fondue, but maybe I really like steak more. It's hard to relax while shopping—still. Good thing I gave up sugar when I got my cancer, because I don't think that I could order my own ice cream. I still sleep on the left side of the bed. The right side is pretty empty.

I am capable of taking out the trash. I have no idea how to turn on the sprinkler system or change the vacuum bag on the central vac. For what cars cost they should just work, darn it. For all I know, the rattle could be one of the grandbabies toys. I still do the dishes, sweep and pay bills, but the only dirty socks I pick up are my own and I don't wear boxers. For me, singleness after couplehood is quite an adjustment. I thought that the first year of marriage was tough, but it's got nothing on the first year of widowhood.

I am a still part of a couple. Steve is gone, but God is here. I know that He is walking hand in hand with me every moment of every day. His promises are true; He will be with me always. He will be my husband and father to my kids. He is compassionate, loving, caring and kind. He is my light in the night and my peace in the day. "The Lord is my rock, my fortress and my deliverer; my God is my rock, in whom I take refuge. He is my shield and the horn of my salvation, my stronghold "(Psalm 18:2, today's verse from the Joy Jar).

God is good, all the time.

March 28, 2009

This was a busy week. On Tuesday I had a visit with Dr. 90210-49503. I picked a pair of implants that will be placed on my body April 24. The round ones felt better than the tear drop shaped ones, so on the recommendation of the great doctor, I chose the round ones. I did complain a bit, on the grounds that women can just buy breasts now, and I have had to wear a bra since 4th grade with no training necessary. And contacts now come in many colors so brown eyed people can now have blue or green eyes or even my color of greenish bluish. Thus, two of my best assets (really three, I guess) can now be purchased by anyone. That leaves me with nice earlobes and pretty good elbows. So far I have not heard of people being able to purchase those. Hopefully, there are some assets I come by naturally that won't ever appear on the menu at the plastic surgeon's office.

Other things that were on the agenda this week: The butterfly exhibit at Frederick Meijer Gardens, condo touring, a great fish fry, an awesome birthday party at Arena Racing, BBQ ribs, Hollywood Rummy and some shopping, or as my nieces say, Retail Therapy.

I did do something a bit off the wall this week (I wonder, is this where the "crazy" starts to show up?). I had another hole put in one ear; a small pink flower way up at the top. It's really cute, but I had to convince LeeAnne (my incredible friend who makes my brother an extremely blessed man) to do the same. She opted for a little diamond at about the half way mark, just as her ear stops folding over. LeeAnne's is really cute too.

I am not entirely sure why we did it. I think it has something to do with her special birthday coming up and my grieving process. Or maybe it was part of her grieving process and I just liked the flower. Either way, we both have really cute ears. Now I think everyone should get their ears double-pierced. It only hurts for a second and is completely worth the pain for beauty's sake.

I miss Steve. But I don't wish him back. I do wish that the circumstances were different and we could be together right now, that he never had cancer, and that I was about ninety five with one foot in the grave so that I knew I would be seeing him soon. But I don't wish him out of Heaven. That would be as bad as giving one of my grandbabies a sucker and then taking it away after just a couple of licks. Right now, Steve is enjoying a really big sucker; a round, swirled kind that candy stores sell but no one ever buys because it would take bus load of people to consume it. I miss him, but I am happy for him. Enjoy your sucker, Babe.

God is good, all the time.

March 29, 2009

On March 8, Steve left his tent behind. The very next day friends came over to participate in a video. Family members, volleyball players, and longtime friends all talked to the camera about how Steve changed their lives.

The video was shown at Steve's Celebration Service. Luke put the video on YouTube. If you would like to view it just go to that website and type Steve Sorrelle in the search bar. You will find "A Tribute to Steve Sorrelle," Part One and Two.
Thanks to you who participated and thanks to you who watch the video. And special thanks to Kelly who put the whole thing together and Josh who made it a little shorter.

God is good, all the time.

April 8, 2009

Today is Steve's one month anniversary in heaven. It doesn't seem like a month has passed since I held him and he held me back. I still expect him to cuddle up to me at night or walk through the door after a hard day of work at the golf course. I am still trying to get used to not thinking about what he would want for dinner or what he would want to watch on T.V. I miss him. But today is a great anniversary, the one of his welcome into Heaven. So today I will be happy for him.

One of the many things I learned from Steve was that expectations can get me into trouble. Our first year of marriage was crummy. It was not what I expected. I would make a glorious meal using a recipe from my new Betty Crocker cook book, expecting Steve would tell me how good the food was, or maybe that I was a better cook than his mother, but he would say nothing. I would work hard to clean our little two-bedroom apartment with no notice taken, no compliment on my wifely skills.

Following an argument, I expected Steve to sleep on the couch and bring home flowers the next day. Yet he refused to sleep in the living room, and the next day there were no bouquets of flowers for me. He also failed to tell me how great I looked after I spent extra time on my make-up and wardrobe choices. His biggest failing was that he didn't read my mind.

During that year it seemed that the more I expected the less he delivered. I was frustrated, sad and angry. Was this guy raised among animals? Didn't he understand how a marriage was supposed to work and what he was supposed to say? I wanted to fight with him, but he didn't even know how to fight. He would fall asleep next to me in bed as if nothing had happened. I would toss and turn, unable to doze off due to my inner turmoil. Steve would sleep like a baby.

Steve, being as astute regarding the emotional mind of a woman as any other man, had no idea I was angry. When I finally reached a point where I couldn't take his insensitivity any longer, I let him have it, using my outside voice to let him know how he has failed as a husband, what he should be saying and when he should be saying it.

Calmly and rationally (I hate that combination when I am mad), Steve explained that he was not at fault, but it was my expectations that got me into trouble. He pointed out that he did not do anything wrong at dinner, but that it was my expectation of a compliment which got me upset. He told me he thinks I am beautiful, and he just figured I knew it. He went on to say that anytime that I expected him or anyone else to act a certain way or say a certain thing, I would face disappointment. Not because the action did not happen but because it did not live up to my expectations. As I thought about it, when the fuming settled down, I realized that he was right. It was my expectations that failed me, not my husband.

Our marriage improved overnight (with both of us in the same bed). Instead of frustration in what was *not* said, I was elated over what *was* said. Each compliment, kind word, and encouragement became a precious gem to me. In twenty nine years I collected a bag full of gems. Steve never really got better at giving lots of compliments, but his touch was my confirmation. The way he would grab my hand to hold everywhere we went, put his arm around me at the movies, snuggle up to me on the couch while watching T.V. and spoon with me in the middle of the night—those things were the greatest compliments of all. He wanted to be near me, always.

Love you, Babe.

God is good, all the time.

April 9, 2009

Expectations, here we go again. Over the years I have thought a lot about Steve's words of wisdom. I have passed his advice on to every new couple I know. But here I am again in the middle of expectations, wondering what comes next.

Some expectations are fine, like expecting the computer to light up when the mouse moves, receiving monthly utility bills and having to bundle up for cold weather in Michigan winters. Some expectations are unrealistic like expecting to win the lotto, believing that your kids are perfect and thinking the IRS will never make a mistake.

For some things it is hard not to have expectations, for example, movie popcorn. When you pay $8.75 to get your movie ticket, and then another $15 for popcorn and a drink, you expect that popcorn is going to be delicious—it had better be delicious!

I'm figuring out what to expect after Steve's death. I had never before held someone in my arms while they took their last breath. I had never had a husband leave this world for a greater one. I had never lived alone, grocery shopped for one, slept by myself for a whole month, had complete control of the remote or shopped for a car for only me.

I don't know if I am doing this "w" (I hate the word "widow") thing the right way. I don't know if I am living up to others' expectations. I don't know if I am acting the way a person in my position should act. I laugh a lot, and I only cry sometimes. My tears seem a bit selfish because I know that they are only for me. Sometimes my tears are not sorrow at all but tears of utter joy for Steve.

༞ ༞ ༞

Time is an interesting thing. Steve told me he believed I would be walking into Heaven right after him. He said that it may be years before it happens, but to him it would seem really soon. I hope so, Babe. I don't know what life will bring. I don't know what tomorrow holds. But I do know I'm not alone, Jesus is my tour guide for my life's new adventures, and God's not done with me yet. God is faithful and His promises are true. He will "never leave me or forsake me." I know that I matter and so does my life if I let it. So here goes. Steve, I promise to make you proud. God, I promise to walk out whatever life you have for me. Lead the way and I will follow. I may not live up to others' expectations, but I sure want to live up to yours, Lord.

God is good, all the time.

April 10, 2009

Chris Tomlin's "Amazing Love" has been saturating my heart today: "I'm forgiven because You were forsaken. I'm accepted, You were condemned..."

God's love is truly amazing, especially in hard times.

Sometimes when I lay awake at night, I think my heart is breaking. To know that whatever God has for me for the remainder of my life will be without Steve is torturous, particularly in the middle of the night. Somehow, even though my heart hurts, it is full and overflowing. God fills the void, the empty space that was Steve by my side.

I have spent the last two nights at home alone. I am capable. I spent many nights alone when I traveled for Careforce International, a Christian humanitarian organization I ran for awhile, and was fearless. I am fearless now, sort of. I have been locking the doors, something that never happened when Steve was here. I guess I will have to locate a house key if I want to lock them when I go out. I don't feel less safe, I just feel more alone.

I have taken out the trash on four Wednesday nights. I don't know why the trash guy did not take the two brown bags of lawn waste that I put by the curb. Hopefully someone will enlighten me. I would just burn them in the back yard, but I think there are laws against that.

I *can* live alone. Or should I say I can live alone, so long as my dad is just a phone call away if I need something repaired. I came home to a fifty degree house because the furnace was not working. Needless to say, my dad was here in a jiffy and I have heat again. It helped that he brought Uncle Bill along. Those two minds have seen and fixed just about everything in a combined 140 years, and they work pretty well together. Uncle Bill has some crazy ideas about evolution, but he can ask God about those later, when he sees Him face to face.

It's Easter time. I love Easter, the yellow marshmallow chicks, black jelly beans, hollow chocolate bunnies with candy eyes, kites, bubbles, and searching for dyed, hard boiled eggs that were hidden the night before. I love getting together with family and shopping for the best Easter dress complete with matching purse, hat and gloves for my granddaughters, my daughter before that and for me a long time ago. I love praying through the Stations of the Cross at a Catholic Church. I weep every Good Friday imagining what Jesus endured. I rejoice every Easter Sunday knowing that He is alive and well, overcoming death and the grave, sacrificing Himself for our failures. For me, nothing compares to the celebration of the resurrection and the celebration of life at Easter.

The Easter celebration in Heaven has to be outstanding. I would love to be that party planner! The menu would have to include something other than the grapefruit and cereal I've been living on. The banquet table, decorated in all of Heaven's finery, with name cards held by porcelain cherubs, the finest, untarnished silver, china so thin it's practically transparent, with beautiful hand painted flowers around the edges, stemware made of the most spectacular crystal, soft linen napkins in a gold and jeweled napkin rings, and centerpieces containing fresh cut flowers that smell as great as they look. The food would prepared by the finest chefs, dishing up delicacies that look almost too good to consume. The dessert table has to be spilling over with chocolates, Tiramisu, apple pie a la mode, my sister-in-law's frosted sugar cookies and yellow marshmallow chicks.

I can almost feel the excitement in the banquet room knowing Jesus will soon be entering. Silence would take the place of conversation at the anticipation of His coming. The doors would open. A bright light would be the first thing seen followed by the first steps of His entrance into the great hall. Applause and shouts of joy would fill the place. Honor and glory and hallelujahs would echo off the walls and ceiling. Joy and love would fill the place. Smiling from ear to ear, Jesus would take His place at the head of the table for He is King of Kings. Let the celebration begin!

Have fun at the party, Babe. Jesus, please give Steve a hug for me.

God is good, all the time.

April 13, 2009

Yesterday was tough, as it was the first Easter without Steve. When I walked in the door at Andi's, I told her I either needed to take a pill or drink a glass of wine. She voted for the wine. I usually have about three glasses of wine each year: Christmas, our anniversary and maybe New Year's Eve. There is something different about Easter wine. Easter wine comes from a box and is served in a water goblet that holds about sixteen ounces. By the time the glass was empty, dinner was over and I think I had a piece of cake. When I looked down I noticed dark brown crumbs on my shirt. Ham doesn't elicit brown crumbs, so I guess I cheated on my new way of eating. I suspect I really enjoyed it.

It was just what the doctor ordered. Wine is supposed to be good for the heart, and this glass definitely was good for my heart.

Today has been a much better, wine free day. I got the most amazing phone call from a woman I am anxious to meet. Premier Cruises gave Family Christian Stores a free cruise to give to a "w". They picked me! I will be cruising the first week of May. The cruise features entirely Christian entertainment like the David Crowder Band and Mercy Me. Mercy me alright! God truly is good, all the time.

As if being blessed with a cruise was not enough, I made a huge discovery while waiting for a prescription refill at Walgreens: sugar free Peeps. That Peeps, the greatest Easter candy ever invented, is now available in sugar free is almost more than I can handle! I have them in the freezer, because expecting them to get stale on their own is just too much to ask.

Praise God from whom all blessings flow! Just when my head was down, He put His hand under my chin to lift it up. God's timing is perfect. I really needed a boost today. The Peeps alone would have done it for me. The cruise is overwhelming.

Things are looking up. I will keep looking up, too.

God is good, all the time.

April 18, 2009

Twenty nine years ago today Steve and I rehearsed for our wedding. All of our bridesmaids, groomsmen, parents, grandparents and siblings gathered at Holy Trinity Catholic Church to run through the ceremony. That night I carried my shower bows taped to a paper plate bouquet and kissed single Steve good night for that last time.

I remember a lot about that day. I remember even more about the next, like taking a bath and shaving my legs, doing my own make-up and hair (before the days of styling mousse), getting dressed at the church and my Aunt Nancy helping me stick bobby pins on my veil. I remember all of the girls lining up in their purple dresses to walk in ahead of me. My dad on my arm, walked down the aisle as if it were the Green Mile. His tears started just before we made our entrance into church. By the time the priest asked who was giving me away, my dad was crying so hard that he forgot his line and tripped over my train on the way to his place in a front pew.

Nothing mattered to me that day except committing to my beloved and starting our lives together. The crying didn't bother me, nor did people coming late or the uncomfortable shoes on my feet. All that mattered was that I had found the man of my dreams and he standing there, looking as dreamy as ever in his dark gray tuxedo with stripped ascot tie.

I walked down the aisle to Annie Eister singing "Sunrise Sunset." Steve and I whispered and giggled through the hour and a half mass/wedding ceremony. We lit the unity candle during "Longer Than" by Dan Fogelberg played on Kathy Jo Misner's guitar.

The 2:00 p.m. ceremony was followed by a 6:00 p.m. reception, a typically Catholic Polish affair complete with kielbasa, sauerkraut, beer and polkas played by a live band (there wasn't this DJ stuff in 1980). We danced the night away, me having the time of my life while hoping I wasn't embarrassing the new in-laws too much.

I remember a lot about not only that celebration but most of the 28 annual celebrations that followed. Our anniversary was special. This year we had planned on renewing our vows. It was Steve's idea. He asked me last November. Of course I agreed, thinking we would escape the fickle Michigan April weather and say "I do still" on a tropical beach during sunset. But Steve had different plans. He wanted family and friends to witness our dedication to each other. Steve wins again.

Steve is not going to be here tomorrow to speak those words again, but our vows have been renewed in so many different ways over the years. The way we forgave each other after fights, stood by each other while battling diseases, didn't care if we could only afford peanut butter toast, loved each other through four kids and four grandbabies, and honored each other through house, job and weight and diaper changes. The vows that we spoke before God on April 19, 1980 were lived out and renewed for nearly twenty nine years.

I love you, Babe. And "I do," still.

God is good, all the time.

April 22, 2009

My dad had back surgery two days ago. The surgery went great, according to the surgeon. Have you ever noticed that a surgeon seems to be the one professional that praises his or her own work? A chef doesn't come out of the kitchen to tell the guests that he did a great job preparing their food. An auto mechanic doesn't say, "I opened 'er up and she was worse than I thought she'd be, but lucky for you I worked my magic." My accountant has never told me that if it weren't for him, I would be paying a lot more in income taxes (although I would like it if he did). But a doctor will come out of the operating room and tell the family just how complicated everything was, but he managed a miracle. Hooray!

Still, I don't like seeing my dad in a hospital bed.

My dad lost his dad when he was nine years old. With three younger siblings to help support, he delivered newspapers before and after school. Before graduating from high school, he joined the U.S. Navy. Each month he would send his checks home to help his mom support his brothers and sister. He ran a mail order business to help his shipmates send home gifts and buy things for themselves, while making extra money for his family. After the Navy he went to Ferris State University on the G.I. Bill, knowing exactly how many Kirby Vacuum cleaners he had to sell each month to pay for rent and food. He met my mom and when they married, he was pulling in forty dollars a week. He soon started his own business, then another, then another with great success in nearly every one of them.

His mind is a computer. He can tell you how many square feet are in a building, how many pounds there are in 238 gallons of gas and how many bags of rice will fit into a forty foot container.

He is a brilliant business man who loves Jesus with all his heart, and his love for family falls just shy of that. My dad believes in hard work and works hard; he's more generous than he is wealthy and gives more than he could ever receive. He cries every time he sees orphaned babies in Haiti and laughs heartily at my attempt at humor (some say my humor is an acquired taste.)

My dad is my hero. Heroes should not be in hospital beds. They should be fighting against injustice, flying in the air and scaling building. Heroes should not wear those nasty gowns that tie in the back and expose one's biscuits. Heroes wear capes and tights and masks and spandex. And heroes don't need Super Hero Surgeons.

That being said, yesterday my dad thought that Truman was president, my nephew was his wife and that he was in Ferguson Hospital (probably because of the lower back pain: Ferguson was known for their hemorrhoid surgeries). Today he is much more coherent and giving the nurses a hard time. My hero is coming back.

I don't know what I would do without my dad. He is my picture of faith, a rock and shoulder on which I can stand. He put up with my teenage years, female hormones and pierced ears ("If God wanted you to have holes in your ears He would have put them there!"). As an adult, for me my dad has always been just one phone call away from an overflowing toilet, broken down car and non-heating furnace.

When God is referred to as Father, I know just what that means. My dad's fatherhood has been an incredible example of a father and a shining reflection of the Father.

My dad, my hero.

God is good, all the time.

April 29, 2009

My dad is doing great. Amazingly, just a couple of days out of the hospital and he has the fire back in his spirit. By the middle of May he will want to be up on a tractor showing his back who is boss.

Tomorrow I'm a leavin' on a jet plane. After a few days in sunny Florida visiting LeeAnne's folks, flea markets and a pedicurist, I will be boarding the Good Ship Lollipop for fun and relaxation. I am so excited for this trip. Between LeeAnne's mom's homemade meatloaf and reading by the cruise ship pool, I think this is about as good as life gets—life here on earth, anyway.

I wonder what Steve is doing. I had a dream he got a job in Heaven's sacristy. In my dream Steve and his dad came back from Heaven. They were both exhausted, not from the travel but just from being here on Earth again. Steve's dad had not yet chosen a job, but Steve was very happy with his. Steve said that Heaven is more wonderful than he imagined and he just wanted to get back there. It was great to see Steve, but I truly wanted him to be able to go back to that perfect place. Who wouldn't wish Heaven on someone you love?

I never thought about there being a sacristy in Heaven. Until my dream I had not heard the word "sacristy" in many years, probably not since I was being taught by the nuns at Holy Trinity. I do love the thought of a sacristy in Heaven, a place where special vessels and vestments are stored. I can imagine

Steve's awe as he selects just the right cloak for Jesus. I can't wait to see Jesus sitting at the head of the table, reenacting His last supper as a man, breaking bread and sharing wine as He tells of His last days. Truly, by His stripes we are healed, and by His wounds we are made whole.

I want to be like Him, to see people the way that Jesus sees them, blind to color, economic stature, ethnicity and educational accomplishments. I want to see people's hearts.

Beyond our hearts, Jesus sees our scars. Jesus does not just see our scars but understands them. He lived through more physical pain than most people ever have to endure in a lifetime, let alone a couple of hours. Being betrayed by those you love has to be the greatest emotional pain anyone ever has to endure.

I have a couple of scars. Scars are worse when they are new, but they do fade. Some scars require Neosporin, and others require a touch from Him. Some scars fade enough that they are hardly visible, while others remain for a life time.

Behind every scar there is a story. The one on my arm is from falling down in a field in the Dominican Republic, while carrying cement blocks. On my foot, there's a scar from the rusty pop can I stepped on years ago, but it's barely there after nearly forty years. Surgery scars from Dr. McAnalogy's handiwork are still dark, but getting lighter. Dr. 90210 promises no new scars on May 13 since he will be cutting into the old ones.

As with everyone else, my scars represent the story of my life. Without scars how exciting would our stories be? It is not so much the scar but the story that matters. Some of my stories may have grown over the years, but the ending is always the same:

God is good, all the time.

May 5, 2009

I am surrounded by water, beautiful, blue, salty water and right now there is nothing more beautiful in the world. I wasn't sure why I was so excited about this trip, but I am slowing finding out.

I met a few lovely ladies last night, also "w's." Michelle from Orlando lost her husband three years ago when two Air Force helicopters crashed off the coast of Africa. Miriam's Bob died about the same time after a three year battle with ALS. Jamie was pregnant five years ago when her Army man was killed by a roadside bomb in Iraq. Kari's Chris, a cop, was on a call while working narcotics when a car pulled in front of his motorcycle last October.

Four wonderful ladies, four different stories. Yet we had an immediate connection. I feel this connection with several people onboard this ship. I keep thinking that I know each person from somewhere. There is such familiarity in so many faces. In actuality, I haven't met these people before, which means to me it must be the whole Jesus thing. Our hearts are connected even though we don't know each other. I believe what I am experiencing here is a foreshadowing of relationships in Heaven. We may be strangers now, but in Paradise we will know each other.

A "w" friend of mine told me that she reconnects with her husband when she is praising God. Her honey moved on to greener pastures a while back and is enjoying life in Heaven with Jesus and Steve. During times of worship filled music, she reaches her hand up, he reaches down and together they sing.

Last night I sang with Steve, David Crowder, Fee and New Day. Mostly, I sang with Steve. When I reach up toward Heaven, I can feel his hand in mine, just like I used to feel it, praising God, loving God and loving each other.

God is good, all the time.

May 11, 2009

Finally, the expanders are coming out and the beautiful, soft, round, squishy, 700 ml saline-filled implants are going in. Dr. 90210-49503 will again work his magic at about noon on Wednesday. Please pray for the great doctor and for great results. It sounds strange to ask for prayer for that area of my anatomy, but hey, they are what they are. Either way, thanks for the prayers. (No laying on of hands necessary.)

I'm still reveling in the cruise. Everything about it exceeded my expectations. From David Crowder to David Nasser to 33 Miles and Mercy Me, the ship was rockin,' and God was praised. As for the food, escargot in garlic butter, roasted lamb, prime rib and grilled prawns were always followed by a sugar-free dessert delivered to the table by terrific service staff. Indulging in a 90-minute spa treatment was pretty darn good too. But the best part of the cruise was the people. I met some wonderful folks I hope to know for a really, really long time.

No matter where, no matter when, how or what, it is the "who" that tops everything. I don't remember exactly *where* I went on a cruise with friends several years ago, but I remember laughing uproariously with them at dinner each night. I don't remember exactly what I bought at Disney World when my kids were young, but I remember meeting our friends, Fred and Mary Ellen, for the very first time on Mickey Mouse's bus.

The friends I made this trip were pretty special. I will remember them for a lifetime and look forward to introducing them to Steve someday.

LeeAnne, by the way, makes a great travel partner. She even sang me to sleep with her Ambien-induced version of "The Old Rugged Cross." I am fortunate to have her and I hope God fulfills her desire for a great singing voice in Heaven. Right now, however, although the sleeping pill didn't do her pipes any favors, I'm happy her voice is still music to my brother's ears!

ৡ ৡ ৡ

Paul prayed for the Ephesians to have the "eyes of their hearts opened." Too often, it's the eyes of our heads that get in the way. A lot of us see people the way the world sees them and judge accordingly. A guy in a suit and tie must be a lawyer or a preacher. The kid with more metal than pimples on his face has to be living in rebellion. The girl with the red, orange and purple hair must be into crazy things like meditation and incense. The man in the pick-up truck wearing a flannel shirt and blue jeans must be the janitor (oops, or my dad).

I learned early not to judge a book by its cover or a man by his clothes. But if I could only live by that every day, to see with the eyes of my heart the way that Jesus sees people, to feel their pain and share in their joys! That is my heart's desire.

My prayer is exactly this, in the words of Paul:

"That's why, when I heard of the solid trust you have in the Master Jesus and your outpouring of love to all the followers of Jesus, I couldn't stop thanking God for you—every time I prayed, I'd think of you and give thanks. But I do more than thank. I ask—ask the God of our Master, Jesus Christ, the God of glory—to make you intelligent and discerning in knowing him personally, your eyes focused and clear, so that you can see exactly what it is he is calling you to do, grasp the immensity of this glorious way of life he has for his followers, oh, the utter extravagance of his work in us who trust him—endless energy, boundless strength!" (Ephesians 1:15-19, The Message).

God is good, all the time.

May 13, 2009

NB Day takes on new meaning today. Yesterday's appointment with Dr. 90210-49503 proved to be fruitful in some ways and not so much in others. Apparently the odds of coming out of this surgery with bull's eyes (I don't want to type the word that rhymes with ripples) are fairly slim. It seems that the new ones have to settle a bit before the things can be centered properly. Although it means an additional surgery, I do feel better about having them head in the same direction. It would be challenging getting used to them if they looked like Marty Feldman's eyes.

This is my first surgery (besides eye surgery when I was 10 years old) without Steve. When he was here, he would always hold my hand and tell me everything was going to be all right. Whether it was a C-section for one of the babies, removal of a kidney stone or a mastectomy, Steve stayed strong while I complained about having to go under the knife, again. He would read to me after the IV was pumped with a little "feel really good now so that you won't run away when we wheel you down to the operating room" medicine. My husband's would be the last face I saw before the big trip and the first face I saw when it was all over. Steve knew exactly where to locate the vomit vessels if I started to turn a certain shade of green. He carefully monitored my pain meds so that shade of green would be less likely to appear.

Steve knew the routine.

Today LeeAnne will be filling in for Steve. I think that she's going to do just fine. She knows me better than anyone and will certainly be able to recognize a color change in my face. One thing LeeAnne and I have in common is that we don't do puke. Either one of us would change a messy diaper, but we do draw the line when it comes to stomach contents. That is where Steve and Joel come in. They are the janitors of regurgitated juice. So, today I will do my best to not let nausea win. I'm sorry, LeeAnne, if I fail.

A nice woman from the hospital just called. Apparently Dr. 90210-49503 is running a bit ahead and needs me to come in early, so I need to go.

I want to end this note with one thought: Love wins,

When all else fails.

When you just can't seem to get along.

When times are tough.

When the hurt is deep.

When the walls are high.

When the kids are rebellious.

When life is crappy.

When you are at the end. Love Wins.

God is good, all the time.

May 19, 2009

I woke up this morning looking forward to the day: beautiful weather, drain removal (see below), and watching Adam and

Kris fight it out on "American Idol." What I didn't anticipate was being reminded again how fragile life is and how each day, each moment should matter.

Dr. 90210-49503, much to my relief, was able to remove the nasty tubing that wrapped around my expensive silicone implants, exited my body through a hole in my side, and led to a little plastic balloon that collected all of the juices that are produced after surgery. The process was not fun but having the drains out is wonderful. I don't remember being so irritated by them after my first breast surgery last October. Today I was happy to know that they were thrown into the trash can and will soon be in the big incinerator to be burned into oblivion, never to hurt anyone ever again.

And the new ones do look marvelous. Round, perky, perfect, a little swollen but truly magnificent; they will forever be standing at attention which is one of the best things that comes out of all of this. The doctor is happy with his work and so am I. Next week I will find out more about the bulls eye construction. I know very little about the procedure. Sometimes ignorance really is bliss. I am thinking that going to sleep without them and then waking up with them, and a couple of Tylenol, will be just fine. I am hoping that Dr. 90210-49503 needs to take some extra fat that I have in supply to form his two projects. Waking up with less baggage really sounds good. I am hoping that someone slips a liposuction machine in the operating room, and the good doctor decides to just go nuts. Oh, the joys of plastic surgery.

After leaving the doctor's office, I received two phone calls nearly back to back that turned my ordinary day into an extraordinary one. The first call was from my cousin, Mary letting me know that a good friend, great mom, and wonderful human being went to go live where Steve lives.

About a year ago Karen was diagnosed with brain cancer. Before the diagnosis Karen was a beautiful woman with an infectious smile. She was a glass half full kind of gal with a heart that matched her outward appearance. Karen loved her husband, adored her kids, and was so proud of them. She never missed one of B.J.'s basketball games or Liz's volleyball games. Stephen kept her smiling and Aaron kept her laughing. Mark was the love of her life, and her countenance lifted every time he walked into the room. Working for Hope Network and helping many people seemed to be her dream job. Karen was a woman who gave more than she could receive, loved completely, and smiled constantly. After her diagnosis she remained true to the person that she was. She kept her chin up and fought with everything that was within her. Through many rounds of chemotherapy, radiation, MRIs, CT Scans, blood tests and more she kept both her dignity and her faith.

Believing for a miracle, Karen was granted the biggest one ever today. This last year has been an all-out war against cancer. Today is an all-out celebration. Good job, Karen, way to finish strong. I am glad that Steve is part of your welcoming committee. You two can share some laughs over volleyball memories from when Liz played, and Steve can tell you some stories about Stephen's trip to the Dominican Republic. You have great kids. They will continue to make you proud and so will Mark.

Then my phone rang again. My dad called to let me know that Uncle Bill had a heart attack, two bad words that you never want to hear together, and never, ever associated with someone you love.

When LeeAnne and I got to the hospital, we found out there was a blockage in his heart which could only be corrected with emergency bypass surgery to save his life. The doctor likened it to the kind of blockage that kills an otherwise very healthy athlete with no forewarning of a serious heart problem. Apparently, if Aunt Barb had not brought him in when she did, Uncle Bill could have been with Steve right now, too. We were able to see him before they wheeled him down to the operating room.

During Uncle Bill's surgery we were thankful to the Meijers for their state of the art heart center, to Aunt Barb for insisting on making the trip to the hospital, and to God for not being done with Uncle Bill yet. There were plenty of tears that came when we thought about what could have been, and plenty more when we recognized the miracle that happened. The projected five-plus hour surgery took less than four hours. The doctor came out of the operation happily optimistic for a full recovery. Aunt Barb gets to keep her boyfriend for a while longer, and we all get to enjoy the fun he adds to our family gatherings.

Two miracles happened today, two really fantastic things. Karen went to Heaven and Uncle Bill gets to stay on earth. To bear witness to both made me realize that people are not just created for God and to bring Him glory, but we are created for each other, too. Each person we meet, everyone that we know, brings a different slant on life, a new view of our existence and our purpose. Karen showed me how to forgive people, not live in bitterness, but instead embrace life for the joy that it has to offer. Uncle Bill taught me what it means to truly love your spouse and live your life to honor your family and

God. Two miracles, two great people. Love you, Karen and Uncle Bill.

God is good, all the time.

May 23, 2009

I am healing. I feel better every day. The first few days out of surgery all I wanted to do was sleep. Now being awake feels great but a nap in the afternoon would be nice. I welcome bedtime, but I always have.

I'm trying to get used to wearing the over-the-shoulder-boulder-holders again. I have gone months without the need for one and thought that I would spend the rest of my life that way. Unfortunately, to assure proper healing, I need to wear the very thing that was burned in the 70's during the women's liberation movement to give us so much (like the right to work 50 hours a week, bring home the bacon and fry it up in the pan, clean the house, dishes and dirty diapers).

I guess it will help to keep the newbies in place. I am all for them staying where God designed them to be. It is bad enough that I have one lazy eye that likes to wander when I am really tired. I do not need other parts of my anatomy facing in directions other than forward.

In the mail yesterday, I received a well-intentioned flyer from a widowed person's group. It was more depressing reading the literature regarding widows than living the life of a widow. Maybe I am just still in the "fog" that is the after effect of loss.

The words used in the flyer included guilt, helplessness, despair, hopelessness, emptiness, and loneliness. The words that would be in *my* flyer would include hope, peace, joy, mercy, love, and GRACE.

Hopefully, I'm not in a fog that will someday lift and leave me unprotected from the grief and bad feelings. Instead, God *is* the fog and He will never leave me unprotected.

❧ ❧ ❧

I've been thinking about what it takes to coach a team to a championship. You start by getting the players into great physical condition: they run, jump, squat, run, lunge, and run some more. At the end of conditioning they are broken and spent, kind of like how I felt when I realized having a relationship with Jesus was the only way of getting up and moving forward.

It's also important for the coach to be reviewing and teaching the basics of the sport. Even if a player has heard it all before, being reminded of the basic skills helps even the best athletes improve. In my early days as a follower of Jesus, I could not get enough of the basics, and even now I love to hear different thoughts and perspectives on anything to do with the character and teachings of God. In sports, tougher skills and plays are added as the season progresses. Stronger competition makes the team better. The toughest of trials lead to the biggest growth in the players. The same thing is true in one's spiritual life.

The big championship game is always make it or break it time. After months of practice, learning, developing, growing, you feel prepared going into the stadium to face your toughest opponent ever. The most important element is to keep your eye on the prize and finish strong. The goal is the same for every team entering into the tournament. The goal is to win. In the same way, every follower of Jesus dreams of the day when they are surrounded by Heaven and the presence of God.

Steve entered the championship game poised and ready for victory. He knew the basics and even a few extra trick plays that kept the enemy off guard, plays like humility, compassion, love and joy. When he stepped out on the playing field, he felt like the season passed more quickly than it should have, but he was ready nonetheless. The final buzzer sounded and Steve won! The trophy was surely bigger than any treasure ever imagined and the reward greater than one thousand of the greatest victory celebrations combined.

Knowing that Steve has the victory, how can I despair? Do the other teams begrudge the champions, or does it make them work harder seeing how sweet winning is? A good coach will bring a team to the next level so they are ready when their time comes. I have the greatest Coach of all. He is getting me ready. I pray I never forget the basics as I grow in knowledge and love of God. I think that my championship game is a ways away. But however long the season is, I just want the coach to keep putting me in. I am playing to win.

God is good, all the time.

May 25, 2009

Happy Memorial Day! Thank you so much to everyone who is serving or has served our country in the military. Thanks Dad, Luke, Noah, Matt, David, Adam, Joel and everyone else who has played a role in protecting our freedoms, such as freedom to share our opinions and hearts, to serve our God, and to be who He has created us to be.

One of our volleyball players from a few years ago wrote to me right after Steve stepped into Heaven. This is what she shared:

"I wanted to say something today in honor of the dozens of volleyball players that Steve and Kim coached at Trinity Christian School over the years. They committed so much time and effort to these teams, and have made a huge investment in so many lives through this. As I share a small piece of how they impacted my life, I know this could be multiplied dozens of times over for all the teams they have coached through the years. When I entered my freshman year at TCS, I was tall, awkward, and shy. When the varsity team needed a middle blocker, they could have easily found girls more talented, but being at least eight inches taller than my classmates, I was drafted to Kim's team. Over the next four years, I spent many after school hours at practice and games with Kim and Steve.

Even while at practice, you could always see their adoration for each other. Kim would frequently look at Steve across the gym and say things like "Isn't he cute?" Steve would respond with his big smile and make a joke like, "Well that's why you married me isn't it?" You truly knew that they were still crazy about each other.

When I knew them, they lived in Grandville and had a weight bench in their basement. My sister and I spent many, many evenings at the Sorrelle house lifting weights, and Steve always volunteered his time and effort to design our workouts. He taught us how to bench press, squat, and I know that my scrawny arms could not have been able to hit the ball as hard without those many hours in the basement lifting weights surrounded by volleyball posters and inspirational quotes. Later they put a spiking apparatus in their backyard, and always had the doors open to come work on lifting or volleyball.

During the season, we would often meet as a team at their house before and after tournaments. They would feed us muesli at their house in the morning, load us all up in the Suburban for tournaments, then spend all day Saturday coaching, cheering, encouraging.

When it came time for me to go to college, Steve took time to put together a tape for me to send to colleges, and Steve and Kim came to see me play when I would have tournaments in Chicago.

I didn't completely appreciate then what a sacrifice and tremendous heart of giving this represented. Despite both of their busy schedules and work and raising four kids, they took time to invest in lives around them. Now that I am working full time and trying to raise two kids, I feel at times I can barely muster up the energy to invest in those closest to me, not to mention reach out to those around me with such generous and selfless enthusiasm. Kim and Steve were blessed with financial resources, and could have easily turned in to themselves, buying more, spending their weekends golfing (okay, maybe not in December) or helping advance their outward status. But instead they gave their time, their love, themselves.

Really, God was at the heart of all the practices and tournaments. Steve and Kim wanted us to be our best in sports, but more so they wanted us to know God. We always started practice with prayer, talking about God, about listening to him, praying about issues in our lives – and when you have 12 high school girls together, there are always issues.

After high school I moved away to college and didn't keep in close touch, but when I came home for the summer they made a place for me at English Hills to have a summer job.

And when I graduated from medical school last spring, I got a big box in the mail with a giant bouquet of flowers from Steve and Kim.

The picture of Steve that I will remember in my mind is of a man who was eager to smile, to help out, and who liked to laugh. I remember him as a man who spent so much of his life helping others to accomplish their goals and develop into stronger people. He adored his kids and Kim and treated her with so much love and respect. And he had a sincere love for God, and for others to know Him.

Thank you so much Kim for sharing your husband with me and so many others. You and Steve are a living example of what it takes to give from your heart to help others.

Dr. Elizabeth Vanse Martin

Thanks so much Liz. We love you too!

God is good, all the time.

May 29, 2009

I have a big mouth. But I can keep a secret. There have been times when I have not shared things with other people because I was asked not to or it would have been inappropriate or gossipy. But when it comes to my own life, my own stuff, I have a big mouth.

When I was in high school, I went out on a date with a guy from a school in my area. He was a really nice guy and a true gentleman, but after spending a couple of hours with him, I knew that this would be our only date. I did not feel that high school magic, no butterflies in the stomach or little birds singing in the air. On our way home, my date told me that he had a great time and would like to see me again. He then told me that he needed to tell me something before I heard it from someone else.

What? Who says that? The phrase *I need to tell you something* sends chills down my spine. People only use that phrase when something shocking is about to be revealed. *I need to tell you something. I ran over the pet rabbit with the lawn mower. I need to tell you something. Your son fell and hurt his head on the playground and is now throwing up in the trash can. I need to tell you something. We amputated the wrong foot.* It seems like the sentence following *I need to tell you something* might be something someone needs to tell but is also something I do not want to hear.

The next sentence my date uttered was, "Sometimes I like to wear women's clothing. *I* liked to wear women's clothing too, but it's not something I want to have in common with a date! I could have gone my whole life without knowing that information about that boy and survived just fine.

I was mortified. I determined right then and there that I would never tell a soul. I was the first person I knew who dated a cross dresser. I did not even know any cross dressers until that moment and certainly no one in my life knew any, so I was not about to spill the beans and let anyone else in on my little secret.

When he dropped me off, I walked quickly inside, and told my brother and his date that my date told me he likes to wear women's clothes. I made them pinky swear not to tell anyone, ever. There, it was off my chest. I walked across the street to where my parents and several of their friends were playing bridge. I had to let them know that I was in before curfew and that MY DATE LIKED TO WEAR WOMEN'S CLOTHES! Of course, it did not stop there. At school on Monday I told my basketball team, coach and some other friends.

Like I said, I have a big mouth.

I recently made a new decision that I was not going to tell anyone except LeeAnne. Then I decided I would have to tell my brother and my kids. Then if I was telling my kids it was all right to tell my brother's kids. Of course I needed to tell my Dad and Joanne. Now, I am telling you, because I have a big mouth.

On Monday, June 1, I am having what will hopefully be my last surgery for this whole cancer deal. The surgery will give me a look, chest-wise, that will say *It is a little chilly in here but not too cold*. My girls will forever be in an erect position, but not to the point where I will look like a deer in the headlights. Three months from now will be the tattooing.

Now, *I have something to tell you*. I decided to do a little elective surgery since I will be under the knife already and doctors give discounts when you have more than one procedure at a time. I am going to get removed what Dr. 90210 refers to as the "apron" of flesh left in my lower abdomen after the babies were delivered.

I have never had a flat stomach in my whole life. I went from baby fat to "pleasantly plump," as Annie Eister called me. I can't even imagine what it is like to have a flat stomach. I never even considered a tummy tuck before. But I have to say, I am so excited!

There are a lot of really good reasons why I shouldn't be doing this, but none of them seem to matter right now. I feel like I am waiting in line to ride the Magnum at Cedar Point; really excited and really nervous but more excited than nervous. I am going to get into that rollercoaster car and see where it takes me.

I have been riding that rollercoaster for a while now. Life's ups and downs can be crazy. I am ready to see what God has next. I am ready to change the world. I am ready to do whatever it is God has me to do. Lord, lead the way and I will follow. I am excited to see what the next phase of life is, and I am excited to do it in smaller pants.

God is good, all the time.

June 10, 2009

In the last week, I have slept more than I've been awake, tried to live in a no-laughing zone, and left the comfort of my La-Z-Boy just long enough to use the bathroom.

The double whammy surgery, beautifully performed by Dr. 90210-49503, added two small cylinders to the front of me and removed five-and-one-half pounds of "apron." I have a new belly button, an "inny." I am considering getting it pierced when all of the healing is done (the naval, not the cylinders.)

Yesterday was a follow-up visit. Everything is going as planned. The healing takes about six weeks, with another six weeks until the tattooing.

I also visited the great and beautiful Dr. Caughran yesterday. So far the cancer is staying away, and I don't have to go back again until December. It is always great to see her.

I am extremely blessed with the doctors that I have. Somehow, by the grace of God, I have ended up with the best oncologist surgeon, greatest plastic surgeon with the most fabulous nurse in the world. Not to mention Dr. McAnalogy, who did an incredible job with the removal of my lady parts.

I can't wait to go shopping. I am hoping to be in single digit number clothing, maybe even the kind that are always on mega sale since there are only so many buyers for those clothes. The mega clearance racks start at size zero and move up to size eight, then something very scary happens. All of the clearance clothes available in size 10 and above are Halloween outfits, tent dresses and tee shirts that say "My other body is a size 2."

The single digit clothes are cute, contemporary fashions, often marked down 80% below retail. The double digit-ers are clothes that Grandma Hentig would have worn, with the pants never matching the top and a scarf of a different color thrown in to hide any turkey waddle in the neck area.

Really, it's all part of the beauty of being a woman. We can have our own style, way, and individuality. Men basically wear jeans and shirts. We get to wear skirts, skorts, tops, blouses, capris, pedal pushers, slacks, jeans, skinny jeans, relaxed cut, boot cut, flares, shorts, short shorts, in every color of the rainbow. We can choose from empire waist, low waist, high waist, V-neck, scoop neck, button up, cardigans, saddle shoes, penny loafers, stilettos, flip flops, tennis shoes, sneakers, clogs, Birkenstocks, jellies, prairie skirts, mini shirts, pencil skirts, halter tops, spaghetti straps, tank tops, vests, boots, boots in every color and heal height, scarves in any season, hoodies, smock tops, elastic waists, button flies, zippers and snaps.

Oh, to be who we want to be without caring what anyone else thinks, to dress for comfort and fun, to be feminine and tough at the same time, to give more than we get and enjoy every minute of it. I may not be ready for the red hats and purple dresses but I do admire those who sport that look.

God in all of His wisdom knew that two sexes were better than one. I am happy to be a woman and happy that men are men. Where I lack, a man picks up the slack. And fortunately for men, they have us to pick out their slacks. It's like we are two puzzle pieces. Alone, a woman or a man is a great work of art, but fit together, unbelievable beauty comes from the union of the two parts.

So here's to men and to women and our strengths and our differences. And here's to God for creating our uniqueness and our likeness.

God is good, all the time.

June 12, 2009

I had an interesting conversation with Steve's mom yesterday. She said she knows that Jesus said "Ask and you shall receive," yet she asked for Steve to be healed here and instead he was whisked away to Heaven. What she said is true. The words of Jesus are repeated more than once in the New Testament. He clearly says to ask and we will receive, knock and the door will be opened to us, seek and we will find.

How is it then when we ask, the answer we are given is not the one we asked for, and the door opened is to someplace we never even dreamed of? Why is it we seek and seek with everything we have and when we find the answer we have been looking for, it doesn't even resemble the question we asked?

Living a life pleasing to God can end up causing more harm than good to those around us. If we work hard enough to find the faults of those around us, our own faults seem to magnify. Why is it we so easily see the bad in others and even question God's wisdom, yet it's hard to recognize the goodness in people and the true wisdom of God?

What if, instead of seeing the faults and ignorance of other people, including or especially those closest to us, we saw the goodness, kindness, generosity and love they are trying to show others?

What if we could see the world as God does? To see not a world of hatred, pain, despair and degrading remarks toward one another but a world of hope, love, giving, trying to please, and working to make a better world for our children and grandchildren?

What if, instead of being each other's biggest critics, we became each other's biggest fans? Instead of looking for others to fail, we applaud their attempts at success? Instead of tearing apart someone's outward appearance, we recognize the beauty of the heart?

What would our world and our relationships be like if we realized that every single person from the most successful businessman to the hardened criminal, from the single mom just trying to get through each day to the Real Housewife of New Jersey moving into her new mansion, is a child of God, created in His image, loved by Him?

What if, instead of life being a competition, we focused instead on how to have a heart that is longing to be like Jesus, a heart that does not judge someone by what they drink, how they make a living or what clothes they wear, but a heart that looks inward first and foremost to Jesus?

The truth is, God has been at this God thing for a really long time. His experience is unparalleled by anyone, and His wisdom is incomprehensible. For us to ask something of God and assume that it is the best possible thing for us, speaks of our ignorance and arrogance. When we have a question on a business matter we search out the best business mind we know to get advice. His advice might be different than we anticipate, but following it is probably much smarter than doing things our own way. In a medical matter we look for the best doctor in the field to diagnosis and offer solutions. Even if we get a second opinion, it is still some doctor's wisdom that we follow. If a child asks for ice cream for breakfast, but we give him scramble eggs instead, how much more will God's answers to our requests be best? His best might not line up with our perceptions or wishes, but it's still better than our best could ever be.

There are no fancy words or poetic sayings to gain some special place in God's heart. Just ask and you shall receive, seek and you will find, knock and the door will be opened, to His way, the best way.

God is good, all the time.

June 19, 2009

My tummy tuck was a success. I have a new belly button and do indeed look a bit chilled. I am still in recovery mode but getting stronger each day.

The first week after the surgery, I wondered what I was thinking. A tummy tuck, *seriously*. I am 47 years old! Now that I am nearly three weeks out from surgery, I look marvelous. The top of me sticks out farther than the middle of me which is the way it should be, but hasn't always been for me. I am bruised and sore and loving it. When I saw Dr. 90210-49503 last Tuesday I told him that the outside of my upper thighs hurt really bad and thanked him from the bottom of my heart. I wish I could get one of those liposuction machines at home.

By the way, I love the great doctor's staff. His wife is wonderful and I want to hang out with Nurse Joanie. Every one of those ladies in that office is compassionate, efficient and funny. I wonder if he is hiring and what the benefits might be.

༄ ༄ ༄

My granddaughter, Aurora, is a Drama Princess. She called me the other day during a "time out" (something I used to use as a volleyball coach to motivate and reorganize my team, which has now become the preferred method of discipline for children). She *called me.* She is three years old and knows how to use her mother's cell phone! Her texting skills need some work but dialing and pushing "send" seem to be pretty easy for her. The reason for her time out: She "threw a big fit" because she was really needed at work that day, in her mind, and Mommy said they were staying home (she goes to work with Amanda quite often).

There was a bit more thrown into the conversation, in between deep heaving sobs about how Mommy doesn't always understand her, and her life is pretty complicated with trying to fit in tea parties, keeping all of the Littlest Pet Shop pets fed, and finding out what Sponge Bob is up to. She could barely get it all out, being under all of that stress! No wonder she threw a fit. Poor thing, being three years old is not all it's cracked up to be.

According to my brother, Joel, Aurora being the Drama Princess makes me the Queen Mother. As I watch Aurora become Aurora, I feel like I am watching my daughter's childhood all over again.

Amanda was all about the drama. One of her greatest childhood accomplishments was being cast in a starring role in the Tri-unity North Elementary School Christmas Play as Mary, a spoiled little rich girl who wanted everything for Christmas and only got the lead in the play because her daddy bought a new sound system for the school. Talk about type casting. Amanda did not have to do any practicing. She was a natural.

Joel thinks watching Amanda grow up was like watching *me* grow up all over again. I am only one year his junior, so I don't think he can begin to remember what I was like at three years old.

The problem is, I don't think Amanda is anything like me. Alright, maybe she's a little like me. We both have the same walk, or strut, so I am told. We both love volleyball, although I kicked her off the team as many times as she quit while I was coaching her. But we always made up within a couple of hours. Plus, she was the best setter I ever had, and I had some really good ones, so I really needed her. Besides our love for God and each other, I think that's where the similarities end between me and my girl.

It's funny how people see us differently than how we see ourselves. I wonder what it would be like to live as someone else just for one day and see myself through their eyes.

Perceptions are funny things, from what we see when we look at ourselves in the mirror to what we think of our personalities, idiosyncrasies, foibles and humor. For example, my niece Lindsey has a wonderful figure any woman would love to have. She thinks her thighs and upper arms need help.

Luke's wife, 100-pound-Megan (who is beautiful), thinks her stomach is flabby. Lee Anne, who does everything for everyone and would truly give her shirt off her back (if she had something to cover up with quickly), is always thinking she should be doing more to help. Sheila, who I aspired to be in high school and still hope to be when I grow up, told me that she aspires to be me.

So who are we really? I hope when all is said and done, with each passing day, I am who God created me to be. I want to live up to His expectations. After all, what He desires for our lives should be all that matters.

After all, very few people are happy with their exteriors, and of the ones that are, only three are women! Our exteriors are so inconsequential yet a lot of the time it seems more important to paint the outside and never clean out the refrigerator, if you know what I mean.

As I think about my life ahead, knowing it will never be the same as the life that is behind me, I want to look forward to a future uniquely designed especially for me. A future not only full of adventure and surprises, but one that is pleasing to God. A future with clean refrigerators and closets would be good.

God is good, all the time.

June 22, 2009

Today marks three weeks post-surgery, and on a scale of one to ten, one being Quasimodo and ten being Sister Bonaventure, I am an eight. Every time I see a reflection in a store window I wonder who the woman with the flat stomach is standing next to me. Thank you Dr. 90210-49503!

I had the great fortune to spend Father's Day with my son Luke, his wife Megan and two of the most wonderful toddlers in the world, Crichton, three, and Evayah, two. Luke is in the final stages of his education and training to be a nuclear engineer in the Navy. His schooling is in Saratoga Springs, New York. I felt bad leaving my other kids behind, especially since this is their first Father's Day without Steve. I called them all and found out they had made plans to spend the day together. I was so thrilled to hear it. They are all adults and working to help each other, and as a mom, there is hardly anything as rewarding as seeing my grown-up children liking each other. There were days when I wondered if that would ever happen. Let's just say I'm glad the three boys and the girl made it through childhood with their lives and limbs intact.

At 10:00 pm., the day before Father's Day, Megan and I were so excited to find an actual fisherman shopping in the sporting goods department at Wal-Mart, since Crichton and Evayah (via Megan) wanted to buy fishing equipment for their Daddy. We got great advice on what equipment to purchase. Since neither of us knew one reel from the next, and would have chosen a pole based on Luke's eye color, we were very grateful for the information. Armed with the new pole, tackle box and fishing license, we found a place on a river to cast away. Crichton used his Transformer (robots in disguise) fishing pole, while Evayah had fun with her pink princess pole, a fisher-girl's dream.

We stood on a vacant dock, Luke with his beautiful new pole, excited to see what we were going to catch. Luke got his pole ready, feeding the fish line through the hole things on the pole, attaching the new hook to the end, adding a pretty new bobber a couple of feet up the line, ready to catch our supper. It was then we realized there were no sinkers. Luke grabbed his key ring and located a key that he had no real use for, and tied it on to the end of the line to make the hook go down into the water.

After solving the sinker problem, we realized we had no bait. Being miles away from any store caused us to improvise and use lunch's leftover chicken fries. Apparently fish are vegetarians because we did not get a single bite.

Fishing is new to us, obviously.

It's tough to do anything unequipped. People can tell you what to do or what to expect. Books are written on "how to" pretty much everything. With the internet, instructions are just a click away. But some stuff just can't be put into words or even picture guides. That's what I'm finding now. Even though there are some great writers and a plethora of information available on losing a spouse, making it through cancer, what to do when the man you adore went to Heaven without you, and on and on. But everyone is different. Every circumstance is different.

I have found one Author that understands me completely and one Book with lots of answers. This Author's "How To" Book includes ways to have peace in the middle of a storm, joy that is more than you ever thought possible, love that envelopes like a blanket, and life, though full of challenges, rewarding and full.

Jesus, the author and finisher of my faith, my friend, has had a book on "The New York Times" best sellers list longer than any other book. It's a really good read, and I highly recommend it. It even has a part on fishing, which I should have read before we went to the river without any worms. Next time, I will know better. If I could just remember to always use His reference book before I did anything, life would be a lot simpler (or at least less complicated, plus I would probably catch more fish).

God is good, all the time.

July 6, 2009

What a beautiful weekend! I went with my kids to the "Best Fourth in the North" in Fife Lake, Michigan. It has been an annual tradition for the last several years for my kids, and last year I joined them, so now it is my tradition too.

I am feeling pretty good nearly 100% of the time; well, maybe 85%-ish of the time. I do get to add urologist to the number of doctors that I will visit regularly for a while. Last January when I had my lady parts removal surgery, Dr. McAnalogy discovered a polyp on my bladder. Last week I finally met the urologist that was pulled into my surgery after the discovery. The pathology report came back with a "we don't know." It might be cancer, it might not. So I will be internally scoped every six months for a few years, then annually for a while after that. My body sure knows how to have a good time.

ℛ ℛ ℛ

I liked being married. I started dating Steve at seventeen, married him at eighteen and now I am single, after nearly thirty years of un-single. I have been working (sort of) for about one week now. I like working. I have been working for years, so working is something that I really enjoy doing. It is the coming home to an empty house that I am not used to.

Steve was a homebody. He would have rather been home than anywhere else in the world. I, on the other hand, enjoy going out with friends, tripping the lights fantastic. So we compromised and mostly stayed home. After work we would come home and chillax. ("Chillax" combines "chill" with "relax" and is a word my daughter-in-law uses on my grandchildren. They do not seem scared by the word so I thought I would use it.)

In the summer, we might go for a walk or play tennis, but most nights Steve would watch the History Channel, Military Channel or Glenn Beck, while I watched reality T.V. in a different room. There was something very comforting in knowing that while I was entertained by my "friends" (the housewives in New Jersey, Orange County or New York) or rooting for my favorite singer on "American Idol," Steve was just a holler away, and by 10:00 p.m., we would be together snuggling in bed. I liked that.

Being single is *crazy*. I know women who enjoy it, but frankly, I like companionship. I am just the marrying kind. I have faith that God knows if I will be called to singlehood, or if there is a man out there who could put up with me for another 30 years. It increases my faith to know that God *could* create two men with that same ability, but I know that God can do anything.

Marriage is a really cool institution. To have that one person who's not only a friend but an intimate one, is a gift. The relationship between husband and wife is different than any other relationship. To know there will be one person who will stand by you, stand up for you and stand with you through thick and thin is an incredible blessing; a true blessing that can be taken for granted.

Sure, men can be smelly and women can be moody, but the relationship should go much deeper than just today. Marriage starts off with a pebble. As time goes by, more stones are added and by twenty nine years Steve and I had a pretty good sized mountain. The good times, the bad, the times I yelled at him, the times I made him mad, holding hands during walks, stealing kisses in the car, all of it adds up.

Whenever I got so upset with Steve that I wondered if it was worth it, I would pray that God would bring me back to that first stone. After I met Steve and fell in love with him (nearly simultaneously), I could not wait to be married to him and live with him for the rest of our lives. When times got rough, I remembered that first love, the butterflies in the stomach, fireworks and romantic music love. Then God would return me to that spot and I would fall in love with Steve all over again.

God is good, all the time.

July 8, 2009

I woke up this morning feeling crummy. My stomach was flip-flopping and the bed felt like a better place to be than the shower. *Ugg.* Just when I'm making strides at being a regular person with regular working hours and a regular life, I get hit with a stomach something.

I crawled out of bed somewhere between Regis and Kelly and Dr. Phil. As I made my way to the kitchen it hit me like a ton of bricks being dropped from the tenth floor: Today is July 8. Four months ago today, Steve started his first day in Heaven. After I realized the date, my body started to feel better, still a bit crummy, but mostly better.

How is it that our subconscious seems to know more that our conscious mind? I remember after my mom died, I would find myself having a horrible day and have no idea why. Then I would see a calendar and realize it was my mom's birthday or some other special day. I have been a bit grumpy on Mother's Day ever since she left; this year was doubly tough.

I have wondered for years why that happens, how a date, a song, a poem could create such emotion without even realizing the source exists.

Some like Christmas or Easter can create happy emotions. Remembering the toys stacked in the living room after Santa's late night visit or searching for those Easter baskets and finding live bunnies in the basement, brings back great memories and really warm and contented thoughts. Ads on T.V. and the kind of candy sold at stores warn us that those dates are coming, but there is no special Peep made to remind me of my mom's birthday.

I have a theory, a belief really. Although we are flesh and blood, we are also soul and spirit. Just as the heart cannot be separated from the body, the spirit cannot be separated either. We are so much more than arms, legs, eyes and a brain. We are more than flesh and more than spirit, but we are always both.

Things we hear with our ears and see with our eyes not only get into our heads and hearts but also get into our soul. When a song plays that we haven't heard in years, somehow we still remember the words. It's not just that great filing system that we have between our ears but something much deeper, more penetrating. You can ask me the state capitols or to recite "The Charge of the Light Brigade," things I used to know, but there is no file left upstairs. But songs not only bring back words but emotions as well. People's names, poems, Bible verses, fright, joy, break-ups—many things go beyond just the brain or the heart and get into our spirit. Because we are spirit with a body or a body with a spirit; either way we are both.

As much as we would like to separate the two sometimes, it is impossible. Like watching something you want to forget you ever saw, or hearing words you never thought you would hear, the effect is lifelong. The same goes for things we show or say to others. To think that my words are forever imbedded in someone's spirit can be a scary thing to think about. I know that my words have not always been uplifting and positive, but once they are out of my mouth they have the ability to remain with someone else. I can recall only a bit of second grade but I can remember things people said to me that cut my heart like a knife. I can also remember incredible words that transformed and redeemed me, and showered me with love.

Those are the words that I want to speak to and about others, words that encourage, show love, joy, happiness, and kindness, words that when emblazoned on a soul can be recalled and stood on throughout life. So many have gifted me with those kinds of words, especially in the last ten months, and incredibly, in the last four since Steve died.

I want to send *you* a word today. God loves you. He created you to be who you are. You are special. You are a gift to the world and I am grateful to know the God who gifted you.

God is good, all the time.

July 18, 2009

This week I danced and played tennis, the best aerobic exercises available. I love to do both but do not necessarily "excel" at either. It just feels great to get my heart pumping and get a good sweat going. I won't print this week's tennis scores, but I will say that sometimes fun beats winning.

I also had the pleasure of attending a beautiful wedding for an even more beautiful couple last night. As Lindsey and Drew stood under a snow white portico created by the bride's father, staring into each other's eyes, vowing to love and stay true to each other until "death do us part," there was no doubt in my mind that those vows would last a lifetime. Two wonderful people joined together, and two wonderful families committing to help see them through. The blessed union of marriage is a beautiful thing.

I have learned a few things about being a "w," such as when you are forty seven and single, it is assumed that you are divorced. Then when someone finds out that you have lost your husband, pity fills their eyes and usually there is an uncomfortable pause, followed by either a quick change of subject or an abrupt end.

I understand, in a way. It's easy to feel uneasy, not knowing what to say, not being able to relate. But really, everyone has experienced loss and changes in life. We all have crap that we go through. I don't think it matters so much *what* we go through, but how we react to it. Not to negate the hard times, but life truly does go on with or without us. I would rather be on the bus than watch it pass me by time and time again.

As I write this, there is a song, *Wait and See*, by Brandon Heath playing on the radio. Here's a snatch of lyrics for you:

There is hope for me yet...

He's not finished with me yet.

That's how I am feeling these days. There is a lot of time left to accomplish the plans that God has for me. I hope that I never give up on wanting to fulfill and hotly pursue His plan for me.

None of us knows what the future holds, but that's part of the excitement of life. Fun surprises around every corner, new faces, and new opportunities all make waking up in the morning doable.

My brother emailed this to me a while back. I don't know who wrote it. I think that it makes a lot of sense:

Happy moments, Praise God
Difficult moments, Seek God
Quiet moments, Worship God
Painful moments, Trust God
Every moment, Thank God

God is good, all the time.

July 30, 2009

Doctor break! This feels so strange but I do not have another doctor's appointment until September 11. It was nearly a year ago that life took such an unexpected turn. Last August, I had a mammogram that eventually changed me physically, spiritually and emotionally. Since then doctors have been a big part of my life. I love my doctors, nurses and their support staff! To think I will have an entire month without seeing my new closest friends does not sound that great to me, believe it or not. How will I know when Joni's daughter has her baby or what is happening with Melissa's kids? I guess I will have to wait until September 11 to see baby pictures. I miss Steve *like crazy*. I have been trying to play more tennis lately, which is something Steve and I used to play as much as our summer schedules would allow. Even though he would beat me every time, I sure would like to lose to Steve again.

Living as a single woman is not all that. Some of my home-owning skills need a lot of work. As light bulbs burn out in the fixtures, twenty feet above my head, strange plants overtake the landscaping and trash gets forgotten on early Thursday mornings, I realize having a handyman around was a real bonus. Steve was great at taking care of the "man" things. He might have only emptied the dishwasher once a month, but I never had to plunge a toilet.

I have decided that some stuff I must learn and other things just won't get done right now. I can live with lesser light in the family room, weeds are just as green as Hostas and I will be careful in regards to my toilet paper usage.

Bomshel recorded a song called "Fight Like a Girl" and it's become my anthem. The lyrics inspire me to take on the world, and "conquer with love," always fighting every challenge "like a girl."

With God's help, I *will* keep fighting like a girl.

God is good, all the time.

August 13, 2009

Tomorrow is Steve's birthday. He will turn 52. Most years I would take Steve somewhere for a few days of celebration. Last year at this time we were in Frankenmuth, Michigan. We stayed at the Bavarian Inn, discovered a great park with turn of the century buildings, went on a paddle wheel boat trip, re-discovered the great taste of Reunite Lambrusco (on ice, so nice) and bought a few Christmas ornaments at Bronner's.

No matter where we were, I loved being with Steve. Even though I had to pack for him, he was still the best travel partner.

I'm not sure what to do with my newfound freedom. The last time I was truly alone, I still had a curfew and emptied the dishwasher when I was told to, rather than because it needed to be done. I was only 17 and a senior in high school.

In my days before Steve, I loved to date. The excitement of getting ready, showering and shaving, trying on eight different outfits, taking extra time on hair and makeup, then waiting for "him" to arrive, made my heart beat faster. A movie, maybe dinner or a party made for a good date. I was not looking for a husband, but have to admit that I liked men, good looking, good-smelling men. Men, who open doors, laugh at my jokes and make me to laugh at theirs. I preferred and still prefer manly men. Not an overly sensitive guy, but a man who knows he's a man. So back in my dating days I liked football playing, arm wrestling, weight lifting, home-coming kings in blue jeans, Adidas t-shirts and English Leather.

Being married to a real man for nearly thirty years has not changed my taste in men. There are new, better smelling aftershaves on the market, but basically men seem to be the same. After not looking for so long, I am not sure about a few things. I used to be a great judge of "good looking," but for years now when someone pointed out "good looking" to me, my response would be "Maybe, but he is no Steve."

Also, I don't know if I know how to kiss anymore. I used to. In fact, I think that I was pretty darn good at it. Now I only know how to kiss Steve. I hope it's like riding a bike.

I have actually been out on a couple of dates. It almost feels like high school again, except that I narrow clothing options down to two before I try them on, and I have hair and makeup down to a science. Now being married—*that* I knew how to do right. It had a little to do with waiting for the commercials to ask questions when the History Channel was on, and a lot to do with choosing to love the one I was with.

I thank God Steve chose to love me too.

God is good, all the time.

August 16, 2009

Celebrating Steve's birthday was wonderful. Paul piloted the boat to a great beach on Lake Michigan, where we ate a picnic lunch Laci had prepared. Aurora swam like a fish and Cordelia loved the water too. Matthieu brought a bottle of champagne from France, and we toasted Steve while reminiscing about not so long ago. I miss you, Baby. You have some really great kids.

ℛ ℛ ℛ

Let me tell you about some special friends of mine, the Kubiaks. I grew up in a great church, living in a great neighborhood where everyone knew everyone. The Kubiaks were one of the really special families in our area. Mr. and Mrs. Kubiak were always smiling, laughing and welcoming. All of their kids were smart, kind, warm and a lot of fun.

Jean Kubiak was a couple of years ahead of me in school. I always admired her wit and wisdom. When Steve and I were first married, we double dated with Jean a few times. I always believed that whoever finally won Jean's heart would be a very lucky man. That extremely lucky man was Roger.

Roger and Jean had two boys with the Kubiak smile and humor. And then they had Hannah, a chip off the old block. Hannah could keep up with the Kubiak clan pretty easily. If eyes are the windows to the soul, Hannah's eyes give her away every time. Those baby blues show joy and compassion with just a hint of mischief. At just fourteen years old, Hannah has strength that anyone would envy, faith that could move mountains and joy that could consume a room. She's the apple of her daddy's eye, the close friend her mother adores, and the pal who keeps her brothers hopping. Hannah is one of a kind.

Last September, Hannah was diagnosed with cancer. Roger and Jean read, researched and sought counsel from the best of the best in the world, while spending time on their knees pleading for a miracle. That miracle came yesterday when Steve helped welcome Hannah into Heaven, where Jesus wrapped His arms around her and made all of her pain go away.

Hannah fought hard. Her parents and brothers were her greatest advocates. The Kubiaks stood strong too. Over the past year, they posted updates about Hannah, and I read about a party at Aunt Mary Jo's, or a Kubiak family get-together. I admire their support, love and endurance. They are so fortunate to have each other.

God puts people into our lives to give us the physical, emotional and spiritual support that we need to get through the tough times, and celebrate with us during the good times.

The Kubiaks will never be the same. They will love each other and appreciate each other even more. They will all miss Hannah like crazy, but they will do it together, united, for each other.

God is good, all the time.

September 1, 2009

One year ago today I met with a surgeon and my world started spinning out of control. One year can change a lot. Life is good, just not as good as it was. Steve always made things better somehow, and he's not here.

Something very significant happened last week. It started out with a fun evening out line dancing with pals. You see, every Wednesday I go line dancing. I find it to be the best three hours of aerobic exercise available. I guess I am just a good ol' girl having a good ol' time. I meet up with my line dancing cousin Cheri, and friends Elsa and Kimberly, so we can drive to The Barn together.

On the way home last week, Kimberly's left rear tire completely flattened. It was very dark (and probably foggy and rainy and creepy), and nearly midnight when Kimberly pulled over on the expressway in the middle of nowhere.

As we sat in the car debating our future, I confidently claimed we could change the tire. *Yeah, right.* I had never changed a tire in my life. That is a man's job which is why I have a man for a dad, and had a man for a husband, then birthed three sons. Men change tires, mow lawns, take out trash, shovel the driveway and take naps on Sunday afternoon, not women (or, not me).

Since it was nearly midnight, I decided that it would be much nicer to let my sons and father sleep than to drive for miles to change my tire. Cheri agreed that "maybe we could do it," so out into the deep darkness we went.

Finding the tire, jack and other tools wasn't too hard. Kimberly knew right where to locate the "pop the trunk" button. After lifting out the spare tire, it was time to figure out how to use the jack—not so easy. Then it was time for the lug nut removal. After we all strained trying to loosen the bolts, I decided to stand on the wrench thingy and jump on it. The other three held on to me so I would not fall and break anything that would prevent me from line dancing that week. It worked. The nuts came off and all of my bones were still intact.

Getting the actual tire off of the car proved to be the most difficult challenge. Cheri and I tried to flag down a passing vehicle, but at that time of night there weren't many cars on the road, plus it was so dark out I don't think anyone could see us. Kimberly put a call into the line dance DJ to stop by on his way home. Knowing help was on the way was comforting, just in case.

After one and one half hours, the tire was changed. We did get a little help from a nice young man who pulled over when he saw us, to get the tire off, but girl power paid off. I am now confident that I could change any tire, anytime, anywhere.

I feel so empowered! I can change a tire. I can take out the trash. I can shovel snow. I can even take naps on Sunday afternoons. With God, all things are truly possible. I am not alone in the dark. He will help me loosen the lug nuts of life. I don't need a lug or a nut because I have Him in my life. Although I wouldn't mind a good lug if God has one for me.

God is good, all the time.

September 11, 2009

Life changes every day. Today is the only day that will look exactly like today. Today a baby will be born, a couple will say "I do" and will never, ever check the "single" box again, "divorced," perhaps, "widowed" maybe, but never "single". Someone will die today.

Today someone will win the Mega Millions lotto, and someone else will break her boyfriend's heart. Today someone will pass the bar exam, and someone else will fail it. Today someone will get a new job, a new opportunity, or will meet that someone special they have been waiting a lifetime to find. This is the day a relative from long ago will be forgiven for a horrible past sin, and relationships will be healed. Life will change dramatically today.

Today.

On *this* "today" eight years ago, life was turned upside down by a few radical men who believed their way was the best way. The security we felt in our country vanished, and the trust that we once had in other cultures and countries left. The loss was felt by everyone. No one in our country was untouched by the incredible devastation. Life changed in one day.

We all have those days. The days that we remember the phone call or the knock on the door that changed everything. The moment that the pregnancy test showed a positive two pink lines, the small box in the large hand containing the beautiful diamond, the sentences that started with "I have some bad news", the men in uniform walking slowly up to the front door.

I remember those moments, those days. On September 19, 1980, a phone call from my brother telling me that my mother had died rocked my world. On September 11, 2001, I wanted to gather my family and flee to Fife Lake, which I perceived as safe. On September 5, 2008, the nurse said the biopsy revealed cancer. On January 16, 2009 Steve called from the E.R. to let me know that there was a mass on his liver.

One day. One moment in one day can put everything else into perspective. Does it really matter if the kids walk in with muddy feet? Can dusting be put off a day if it means that you can take the babies to the park to play instead? Is trash really worth an argument? What were you so mad about? Why haven't you spoken with that cousin for this long?

Praise God there are more happy days than sad, more moments to rejoice than mourn, and more joyous announcements than bad news. There are more days to make amends.

But there still remains just one "today."

Yesterday, I had some cells extracted from this little lump in my armpit. I should get a phone call next week from the beautiful, wonderful oncologist telling me that everything is perfect.

Although I am doing my best not to worry, I have been down this particular road before. So be prepared to rejoice with me when the tests come back negative!

Cherish today. Live today like there is no tomorrow. Rock someone's world today in a really good way.

May the God of peace and love and joy and understanding embrace you today and forever.

God is good, all the time.

September 19, 2009

Good news! The lump under my arm contained no cancer cells. Praise God. I wasn't *really* worried, just kind of worried. It was one of those things in the back of your mind you try to ignore, but yet it affects your thinking without your knowing it. Grieving can be like that.

I have not read much about grieving, nor studied what happens to the person that remains behind when a spouse moves on to the Big Golf Course in the Sky. I still haven't met with any support groups or counselors, and have no idea as to the series of feelings which I am supposed to experience, or in what order.

All I know is that I need to keep reminding myself God is good, my kids are wonderful, my grandkids even better and I could not get through another day without my family and friends.

I have somehow survived six months without Steve. I have learned so much in the last six months, like how to change a tire, how to work the DVR (sort of), and that if the trash cans are not taken to the curb on Wednesday night the trash will not be picked up on Thursday morning.

I don't want to do any of this without Steve. Not that I plan on leaving anytime soon, but I didn't sign up for *just* twenty nine years of marriage. I signed up for the lifetime plan, the whole kit and caboodle, retirement in a warm climate, getting so old together that we would become the crazy ancient couple at the Sorrelle family reunions.

Six months! I don't know if something important happens for everyone else at this point in the grieving process, but I know what has happened to me. It seems to be a lot like my first year of marriage. Here I was at the ripe old age of eighteen and Steve a wise twenty two. The first few months were definitely the honeymoon stage. I was just giddy and glassy eyed to be with this hunka hunka burnin' love. Then something changed. It was like I was a child testing a new babysitter.

Subconsciously, I wanted to test Steve to see how far I could push him, but not push him out. I was a witch but with a "b." I was demanding, obnoxious, rude, crude and spoiled. I got angry at little things, really, I got angry at everything. I had to work all day to bring home the bacon, fry it up in a pan, clean our little two-bedroom apartment and wash his socks and boxers. I wondered if we would ever be able to afford a house of our own or the next electric bill. For several months, I was a pain in the behind to live with, and thought that Steve was silly to stay with me.

But he did. Not only did he stay, but he forgave. He put up with my crankiness, hugged me after I threw a fit, helped a little with the dishes and let me get a puppy. Steve did not let me get away with my behavior. He was quick to straighten out my wrong thinking. He never left our bed to sleep on the couch and he never walked out the door angry. He just put up with me. He loved me through it, for better or for worse.

Throughout the years of our marriage we would joke about year number one. I didn't mean to be this crazed, immature girl. I don't know why I felt like I needed to test Steve's devotion and love, but I did. And he stayed forever strong, patient, and loving, forever Steve.

Now the honeymoon stage is over again. The last six months I have tried to be strong for everyone around me. I *want* to be happy for Steve. I *want* to be what Steve would expect. I want to show a Steve-like maturity and strength, kindness and contentment.

Today, I just can't do it. I am sad, angry, anxious and feeling lousy. I am feeling like that old Buck Owens and Roy Clark "Hee Haw" song:

"Gloom, despair, and agony on me...If it weren't for bad luck, I'd have no luck at all."

Tears seem to come easier now than ever. Sleep evades me (although medicines help). Mornings are really difficult. Going to work each day is hard. Trying to keep up with my house and yard has been impossible. My heart bleeds when I think about spending the rest of my life without Steve.

I need to get my focus clear again. I am praying for eyes that see Jesus in everything, everywhere, all the time, and for bright lights in dark days. I am praying for good news, and that I can figure out what it is God wants me to do with my new, single life. I am praying God takes really good care of Steve. I am praying I can be grateful for the years I had with a great man and not regretful for the years that could have been.

Love you, Babe. Miss you. Have fun mowing those greens in Heaven.

God is good, all the time.

October 4, 2009

Friday was tattoo day. I have had a long time to think about exactly what I wanted. I imagined what they would look like in different colors and designs. For a while I thought round was boring but a flower or star shape might be fun. I contemplated going with my favorite color, purple, or perhaps something that would glow in the dark like a nice florescent green. When Steve and I discussed it, he recommended LED lights pointing out of the middle. So many possibilities!

When I finally decided what I wanted, it made me much more excited about going through the procedure. I settled on a circle of pretty pink with a filigree design around the circle. The way I see it, I will be the only one seeing the tattoos, so I might as well enjoy them. I guess someday they may have a coming out party of sorts, but that would be with someone really special who would know the circumstances behind the artwork. Otherwise, they are for my eyes only, and I will probably show my daughter, my son's wives, my sisters-in-law, nieces, close friends, and … Alright, so I will be showing off my incredible doctor's work a bit! Maybe I should have entered Artprize, because after all, Dr. 90210-49503 is indeed a master artist. Maybe my tattoos and I will enter next year's competition.

Unfortunately my desire to have the most creative pair in town was thwarted by the tattoo artist, who had no sense of humor. Come to find out she only does cosmetic tattooing and does not get into the true art form of body paint. Bummer.

Right now, I have pink circles, sore and swollen. I have to go back in five weeks for touch-ups. I am going to start making phone calls to find a great artist to add some flair.

ℛ ℛ ℛ

I want to stop listening to the news, as I get a pit in my stomach when I hear how bad the economy is, how many people are out of work, who planted what car bomb in which city, and how many years it will take for the stock market to bounce back to where it should be.

When I turn on the radio and hear the constant infighting between political parties, religions (including within the Christian faith), national leaders and people groups, I just want to yell "stop!" What is it changing? Who is being helped?

I am done with bad news, with listening to the constant barrage of sadness, sickness, death and destruction. I am done with the "woe is me" naysayers and bearers of bad news.

I want to hear about the good stuff. I want to hear the stories about the people who got new jobs even better than the ones from which they were laid off. I want to hear about people helping other people, feeding the homeless, taking an elderly person to the doctor or providing someone with a place to stay. What about the couple that just had a baby after trying for years to conceive? How about the twenty-year-old who has just been pronounced cancer free? Where's the hope, joy, and love?

If I could host a radio program, I would want people to call in and talk about the happy things going on, celebrating, enjoying, encouraging, coming-out-shining-on-the-other-side kind of stories. My listeners would call in with uplifting stories instead of defeating ones, helpful not hurtful tales, and joyful rather than painful anecdotes.

I choose joy. Cup half full, food on the table, roof over my head, close-knit friends kind of joy. I opt for deep down, true joy, which barrels through the pain and hard times and rejoices in the happy and good times.

I pick joy that can't be understood or explained, the kind that comes in knowing there is a greater purpose, something, *someone*, bigger than we are. Joy in knowing our existence is not dependent on the stock market or global warming. Joy in knowing we are not alone. Joy in understanding God is on our side, loves us and will take care of us. Joy in life. Joy in love. Joy in today. Yep, joy trumps the alternative. Joy wins!

God is good, all the time.

October 13, 2009

My life has been a bit bipolar lately. Some very happy stories have come my way.

For example, my five-year-old nephew helped a physically challenged classmate climb to the top of the hay pile. A dear friend helps out-of-work, homeless people find jobs and a place to live while showing them love and compassion. A former volleyball player is working hard to help poverty stricken kids living in Mexico City. My sister-in-law received a great job promotion. A few people told me that they are going to stop watching the news and instead hear news from "independent reporters," such as friends and family. There is more joyful news in this world than ever gets reported. I wonder what it would be like if news was reported with a joy slant rather than a right or left leaning?

It's hard to know what to say to someone who bears bad news. When a doctor gives a life changing or life ending diagnosis, words can seem insignificant in the face of an unknown future. Some of the words I have heard over the past seven months have been:

"You need to move on"

"Get over it"

"Life goes on"

Well-meaning people try to help bring me to a place where Steve is in my past and my future starts now.

But Steve will always and forever be a part of me. Steve and I grew up together. We shared children and grandchildren. We shared intimate moments, just the two of us. We shared mortgages, banana splits and socks, weekend trips to bed and breakfast inns, anniversary vacations to Disneyland, San Francisco, Ashville, Chicago and Philadelphia, and surprise birthday parties featuring a guy playing spoons, and tee shirts that said "In dog years I'm dead."

Together, we embarked on family vacations to Disney World and St. Croix, mission trips to the Dominican Republic right after Hurricane George, and New York City right after the attack on the World Trade Center. We divided time managing the remote control (sort of). We shared a bed, blankets and sometimes even a pillow. We shared colds, French fries and volleyball teams, victories and defeats, good times and bad times, sickness and health.

I will *not* "move on," But what I will do is move. I will make myself get out of bed in the morning, put one foot in front of the other and muster up new determination each day. I will not let death defeat me. Jesus came to defeat death so that we could have the opportunity to live, not just beyond life on Earth, but to really live life here, today.

God is good, all the time.

October 20, 2009

As I struggled trying to open a jar of salsa the other day, I realized that what I want for Christmas is one of those rubber things that open jars with no trouble at all. Tomorrow is trash day, so I would also like a trash compactor; then I would only need to haul one bag to the curb each Wednesday night. And a step stool would be nice, because my cupboards are tall and I am not.

I really want a lawn boy too. The guy who mows my lawn does a great job, but I need it edged, weeded, seeded and groomed. Plus the lawn boy could turn into a snow boy. Snow shoveling isn't my gift. Plowing? I can get that taken care of, but what if it snows in the night and I have to shovel just to get to my car?

And, oh boy, I *really* need a plumber. I can plunge with the best of them, and I can even stop the water from flowing out of the toilet. But what if something starts to leak?

I'd like to add electrician to my list, because I have this outlet that only works sometimes. I think there is a switch controlling it, but I really don't know. I could try to flick the switches but who has time for that when *So You Think You Can Dance* is on? Also:

> •A foot warmer. Those Michigan sheets can be pretty cold when I climb into bed. A hand warmer would be nice too. Any car north of the Mason-Dixon Line should have heated steering wheels as part of their standard packaging.

> •A full length mirror that can tell me if I look fat in my clothes. Clothing stores should have those mirrors just

outside of every dressing room, right by the chair where the sleepy, nodding guy always sits.

•A mechanic. There is this noise my car started making. It's sort of a *kaaaaaa* but more of a *chuuuuuu*; could be a grinding with a little squeaking. Whatever it is, I discovered if I turn the radio up loud enough, I can't really hear it anymore. I may need him to determine if I also need new tires. I know there is something about a dime, that if you can put a dime in the treads it means six more weeks of winter, or maybe it's a quarter? I usually put my change in those jars with pictures of sad children by every cash register, so I really can't check my tires, even if I understood how.

My list is getting longer as time goes on, so here goes one more wish:

•A Magic Football gizmo, kind of like the Magic Eight Ball, but in the shape of a football. Instead of asking "Will I find my other sock today?" and get an answer like "maybe" or "not looking good," I could ask, "Why did they just call back that touchdown?" and receive "offensive holding" or "the refs get paid by the home team" as answers. I love football and I know a bit about the game, but sometimes there are crazy things that happen and a new rule gets thrown into the mix. I need that Magic Football to tell me why.

As I look over my Christmas list, I realize that at one time I had everything on my list. I had the jar opener, the electrician and the Magic Football. I even had the lawn boy and the plumber, the foot warmer, the step stool and the snow man. His name was Steve.

Now I have my son Paul, my dad, and my other sons, Luke and Noah, helping me to do some of this stuff. Sometimes salsa has to wait until Noah comes home for the weekend, and none of them watch football but, in general, they take care of my house things.

I have someone else too, my comforter, protector, healer, wisdom giver and friend. When the men in my life are unavailable, God is there. He watches football games with me. We cringe together every time a player gets hit really hard, and cheer enthusiastically after a great play. He makes sure the Boogie Man stays away from my house. God keeps me stable when I climb on the cupboard to reach something up high and has done a great job of keeping the snow away so far this year. Plus, He doesn't tell me if an outfit makes me look fat because He thinks I look good in anything, even sweats.

God is good, all the time.

October 26, 2009

What a week! It was the first anniversary of losing my two greatest assets, and my 30 Year Class Reunion. Neither event brought much emotion, although the reunion did make me laugh.

Life has gone on just fine without "the girls." The tattoos have healed nicely, and the new ones seem to get along just fine. In just one year they have come a long way, baby!

My class reunion was a riot. I have the best classmates of all time and when we get together it is as if no time has passed. *Super fine, '79!*

A couple of them spoke of the day I came to school at the end of our senior year and announced that I was going to get married. No one believed me. Not because I was known for telling untruths, but because I was the picture of independence, destined to be the first woman President of the United States. What man could ever harness such unconstrained liberation?

Apparently, his name was Steve.

Steve and I were really opposites in so many ways. He was a pessimist (he called himself a "realist") and I am an optimist (he said I lived in "La La Land"), Eeyore to my Tigger. I love sports, he loved history. My bags remained packed just waiting for the next adventure; Steve's favorite place was home. Steve was steak and potatoes to my Thai and Tostadas. Steve's words were few, wise and thoughtful. Words spew from my mouth like sunflower seed shells out of a little league pitcher. Steve was blue jeans and a pick-up truck. I am go-go boots and a sports car. Steve enjoyed the symphony, I love rock 'n roll. Steve savored quiet walks on the beach. I want to ride the waves.

Even physically, Steve and I were an odd couple. He was six foot three to my five foot two. He wore size twelve shoes! Moses could have floated down the river in one of his Docksiders. Steve had toes as long as my fingers. He was a long string bean of a guy (as my dad once said), while I have always been curvy (my term, not my dad's). My dentist is a good friend but never listens when I beg him to say those two magic words, "no cavities." Steve very seldom had to have a tooth filled. I am always having problems with some part of my body, while Steve had an occasional sniffle.

We were Felix Unger and Oscar Madison, Abbott and Costello, Lucy and Ricky.

I remember years ago hearing a well-respected family counselor say that opposites attract but should never marry. Even the most revered advisors can be wrong sometimes.

It was our differences that made us so good together. Where I am weak, Steve was strong. When he lacked confidence, I had enough for both of us. When I lacked faith, Steve doubled up on prayer. He was yin to my yang. We went together like "rama lama lama ke ding a de dinga a dong."

It is the same with God. God brings peace in the middle of my crisis, joy into my sadness and comforts my loneliness. His shoes are big enough for the both of us, and He shoulders not just my tears but my woes.

Without faith I am really alone. Aside from God there is no hope. But with God all things are possible and great things are probable.

God is good, all the time.

November 2, 2009

Physically, I am doing alright. I have had a bit of laryngitis for the last week or so, which some would say is a blessing. Other than that I am A Okay. This Friday is "Tattoo Touch-Up Day" at Dr. 90210-49503's office, so I am looking forward to seeing the ol' gang.

Mentally I am foggy, but maybe a little less foggy than before. My fits of rage have subsided a bit, the pit in my stomach is a little smaller, and I am beginning to see the muted lights at the end of the tunnel.

I have questions, so many questions.

When I was a kid, I would dream about what life would be like after the millennium. In my imagination robots would be doing all of the dusting and vacuuming. One push of a button would deliver whatever I wanted for dinner. I knew that cars would fly if someone wanted to travel the old fashioned way.

Otherwise people could be teleported to anywhere in the universe. A stylist robot would operate a blow dryer and curling iron, stopping any chance of a bad hair day. The pictures on the living room walls would change from rolling waves to aquariums full of tropical fish to a spectacular sunset with the flip of a switch. All the lighting and temperatures in my luxurious, sky high mega pad would be voice controlled. The climate could go from a balmy 82 degrees to a "turn on that fireplace" 68 at my simple command.

When the year 2000 came, life would be a bed of roses.

My dream has been shattered. I still do the vacuuming and dusting. The button to have the dinner of my choice is the one at Sonic Drive-In. Cars are still on the ground, and I have never been teleported anywhere (except when I am in a hot bath with lots of bubbles, candles, and my favorite CD). Blow dryers seem to take longer than ever, and according to my brother, I have more bad hair days than good. My pictures remain the same; I have to manually turn on the lights and the thermostat does not have a "balmy" setting.

Not only are the mechanics of life different than I pictured but so are the people. I remember watching Richie Cunningham experiencing his crush on the pretty divorcee next door. She was "hot to trot" according to the Happy Days gang, and to Mr. and Mrs. Cunningham she was bad news, an outcast, no matter the reason for the divorce.

I am now the outcast, and I'm not even divorced.

Once upon a time, "w's" (I am still trying to get used to the word "widow") were taken care of, helped out, admired for their strength. Now, it seems that losing your husband gives you some kind of disease. Statistically, when a woman loses her spouse, she loses the majority of her friends, over half of her income and gains twenty pounds. As if losing your best friend isn't enough.

Fortunately, for me the twenty pound weight gain hasn't happened (yet), so I have caught a male eye or two. The conversations seem always go the same way. The innocent flirting turns into small talk which leads to "Are you single" followed by "How long have you been divorced?" With over 50% of marriages ending that way, I suppose it is a natural assumption. But when I retort with "My husband passed away" the backing up begins. First baby steps, then, before I know it, the male eye is running the other direction.

At first I thought that maybe my breath was bad, or perhaps he just didn't like the gravelly sound of my voice. But apparently my breath was alright for the first several minutes, and I like to think of my voice as sultry, not gravelly, and what man doesn't like that?

I came to realize that the "backwards shuffle" begins right after widowhood is announced. I have a disease, an illness, a dirty rotten secret. I have the plague, the "Widow's Leprosy." With it I can turn off a man faster than Carl Lewis can run. But why?

I have long brown hair, green eyes, and I'm slender-ish with a really nice rack (thank you Dr. 90210-49503). I own a house, a car and have all of my original teeth. I am funny, sometimes. I read. Books! I read books. I have a job, a real job, in Michigan, in this economy. I love to travel, go for walks on the beach and watch movies. I enjoy watching football! And I also like Pina Coladas, and getting caught in the rain.

Not a bad package, until the title of "w" is revealed.

Men are not the only ones running backwards. Being a widow in this day and age is like having the Swine Flu. I am not contagious. I want to let people (men are people, right?) know that I lost my husband, not my mind, and although part of me is gone there is a whole lot more of me left. God is not finished with me.

Everyone has a story and a past that make us who we are today. Without them we would be pretty boring. God is bigger than the "w," and Swine Flu. God carries us through those things, goes before us and follows closely after us. He is compassionate, loving and understanding when nobody knows what to say.

Sometimes it is not what we say, but that we do say *something*.

God is good, all the time.

November 9, 2009

My grandson, Crichton, wants to take the bus to school. He is four years old, can get Mario to rescue the princess, thinks dinosaurs can talk and that his Uma is funny. All he wants right now is to ride the bus instead of having his mom drive him to preschool. He sees the allure of that huge yellow machine and wants so badly to climb into the belly of the beast for a ride through the neighborhood. Seeing the faces of his classmates pressed up against the window, breathing hard then drawing pictures in the fog, gives him confidence that the conveyance is a safe joy ride.

Why can't he ride in that big buggy? Why can't he leave class when the teacher announces the bus's arrival? Why can't he jump off that last step into the puddle?

How nice to have simple requests and simple problems.

There are times when I feel like my problems are pretty substantial. Life hasn't been so fun lately, medically speaking. The thought of losing Steve and dealing with my own health struggles, all inside one year, can daunt me. But then I hear about other people's situations, and I realize I am, in comparison, a four-year-old wanting to ride the bus. My situation is so small and manageable when it compares to the plight of others.

I have a roof over my head, and a car with four tires and a fifth in the trunk. I love my job, my country, my church and my friends. My closet has more clothes than I need and more shoes than I care to admit. I am the proud momma of four wonderful adults, the extremely delighted mother-in-law to three beautiful women and very fortunate Uma to the cutest, smartest grandbabies ever. I treasure my Dominican son and his extraordinary family. I have electricity, running water, a machine to do my dishes and another one to wash my clothes. I can openly display the Bibles that I own and listen to Christian radio twenty four hours a day. I can switch between "Top Chef," "18 Kids and Counting" and "Little People, Big World" with the push of a button. The water in my shower is hot and so is the chicken in my pot.

I am fortunate, favored, and flourishing. I am blessed.

Everybody has their thing. Everyone has a struggle. Everyone has an issue. The trick is in not letting the issue or the struggle define, dominate or determine you but rather you define, dominate and determine the struggle.

When I get down because Steve is gone, I remind myself that if I could wish Steve anywhere, it would be Heaven. When I am lonely, I realize I am not alone. When I am sad, I think about all of the wonderful things in my life. When I feel depressed, I remember how much better joy feels. When I get overwhelmed thinking of the future, I decide to live for today.

The joy of the Lord is my strength. (Nehemiah 8:10)

God is good, all the time.

November 23, 2009

Something hit me this weekend, like a snowball in the back of the head. When people make statements like "she acts like an old grandma" or "that looks like an old grandma's couch", I remember that I am a grandma! But grandmas are supposed to be old, hunched, walk slow and bake cookies. Grandmas' smile all the time, wear wire rimmed half glasses on their noses, dresses with small prints and modest nun shoes. Grandmas have their hair cut short or in buns, and buy Halloween candy on November 1st at half price to give away the next year. Grandmas have doilies, crocheted green and orange throws with matching crocheted pillows, small, fluffy lap dogs named Buffy, and lamps that hang on chains from the ceiling. They have plastic on their couches, plastic on their car seats and plastic on their hair in the shower. In Grandma Land scarves are for keeping turkey waddle necks warm, weekly beauty parlor visits keep locks in order, triple coupon day is a holiday. In their purses, they carry pink wintergreen lozenges and starlight mints.

Thus, I now use as my reference for an old, cookie baking, mint toting lady with a bun in her hair a "great grandma," a woman obviously much older than I. I am hoping the new phraseology will catch on worldwide, so I can ignore all of the stereotypes that obviously can't possibly be speaking of me.

♁ ♁ ♁

Last year at this time, I was post-mastectomy, receiving weekly expander inflations from Dr.90210-49503; sugar free, sore but healing and looking forward to turkey and all the fixings with the Sorrelles, with Steve by my side, grandbabies, pumpkin pie, and the Lions on T.V. What could be better than that?

This year as I celebrate the Thanksgiving holiday in Groton, Connecticut, Submarine Base Capitol of the World my list of gratitude is different. I am grateful for Evayah, who at nearly three years old, is an expert makeup artist, for Crichton's sweet demeanor, Aurora's dramatics and Cordelia's spunkiness. I am grateful for Leo's leadership and his healthy new baby brother, Cristian. I am thankful for pink ribbons and research, for my incredible adult children and their equally incredible spouses, for a roof over my head, wonderful co-workers and peanut butter. I am thankful for great friends, wonderful family and Christmas lights. I am thankful for a dad who can fix anything, a mother-in-law who loves chocolate more than gold, and a God who will never leave my side.

Mostly, I am thankful there is life after death for Steve and for me. As I continue to breathe everyday while putting one foot in front of the other, I laugh easily at the blunders that accompany my foggy mind, and explore a new phase of life with anticipation of all that has for me. Steve is living life to the fullest in a wondrous place with a never ending banquet table. I wonder if he will have turkey or "tofurkey" in Heaven? Pumpkin pie will be on the menu, for sure.

God is good, all the time

December 3, 2009

There is no diagnosis yet for Noah, my son, who's been experiencing stomach pain and discomfort for quite some time.

Noah was the fourth born in the Steve and Kim Sorrelle clan. After experiencing the joys, cravings and weight gain of three previous pregnancies, I knew I was not expecting again. Steve was sure that I was.

After taking a 1986 version of a pregnancy test, I left the house to go grocery shopping. Steve later told me the test was positive, which I scoffed off as a cruel joke. But when my monthly visitor stilled failed to show a couple weeks later, the secretary at my O.B.'s office confirmed my fears. Steve was thrilled by the news. He could not stop giggling, just like Abraham. While he laughed, I cried. Just seven months prior, I had my third cesarean section delivery, which was tough. The thought of a fourth was daunting.

But it did not take me too long to get excited for another baby. Somehow I knew I would be having a boy and that God had big plans for his life. After all, I felt a bit like Mary, not because I was visited by an angel announcing the birth of a son, but because we thought the doctor had made having another baby impossible. I was right about the son, wrong about the doctor.

Noah was an easy baby and a happy-go-lucky kid, except when Mario jumped off the edge before getting to the princess. Not as quiet as my other boys, Noah has never had a problem speaking his mind. The upholder of justice, he always believes that life should be fair. Noah can carry on a conversation with anyone, anywhere, anytime regardless of age, position, or language. Although at times his openness regarding perceived unfair treatment of friends and classmates, his opinions on politics and religion and his willingness to share those opinions was not always greeted fondly by teachers, it is that same determined speech that gained him favor with his officers in the Armed Forces, and earned him the respect of many.

A few years ago Noah attended the wedding of a sister of a friend in Montreal. As a high school senior he was pretty good at recognizing a beautiful girl, and there just happened to be one that caught his eye. Marie Sophie Susie Mercier Lefebvre (a.k.a. Susie) was stunning in her perfect little black dress and matching strappy heals. After Noah headed back to Michigan, the two of them corresponded a bit, but got much more serious after Noah committed to joining the Navy a year later.

While in Paris the following February, Susie said "yes" under the Eifel Tower. That May she said "I do." I don't know who was happier that day; me or Noah. Susie is everything I would hope for as a wife for him and another daughter for me. She is intelligent, fun, caring and beautiful. Noah adores her, and so do I, and so did Steve.

Noah and Susie survived the Navy and are now both students at Western Michigan University. Noah is in the Army National Guard Reserve Officer Training Corp, studying pre-med and hoping that his 3.95 G.P.A. will help him get into med school soon. Susie is pre-law, and beats Noah in grades with her perfect 4.0. Right now, they are both a bit nervous that the turmoil of this semester will affect their grades.

Noah has been suffering with severe abdominal pain for about six weeks now. He has been in the hospital more than he has been in class. After several tests with a couple of more underway, there is no diagnosis. His pain is breaking my heart.

Susie is standing beside him, taking him to appointments, cooking his Ramen noodles and making sure he is taking his medications, all while juggling her full class load and a job.

It's troubling, to have my son be in so much pain and have no answers. But when I looked outside this morning to see the first snowfall, I was reminded of God's majesty and sovereignty. The beauty of the white covering the ground, trees, roads and cars is like the blanket of peace that comes with leaning on God for strength, hope, and wisdom.

By myself, I can do nothing, but with God all things are possible. And knowing I can ask for prayer and my friends will pray, beseeching God with me for healing, peace, an answer, prayer pieces sown into a blanket, a covering, a quilt. That's exactly what I need right now, warmth and comfort, security and coziness.

Thank you, Jesus, for wrapping me in your fleece arms. Thank you, friends, for lifting me up in your quilted prayers. Please pray for Noah and Susie.

God is good, all the time.

December 5, 2009

With great sadness, I must share tragic news in my family. This morning Susie lost her dad. At about 10 a.m., Daniel moved in with Steve. He was only 45 years old.

Susie was a Daddy's girl. Daniel adored his only daughter and glowed when he was around her. His gentle heart and quick laugh made him a joy to be around. Daniel did everything he could for Susie. He was even taking English classes so he could communicate better with his American son-in-law. Daniel was kind and loving, compassionate and caring. On vacations to the Dominican Republic, Daniel and his wife, Joanne, would bring candy, pencils, toys, and clothes for the children in the poor schools near their vacation resort. He was great at Pictionary, wonderful with Susie's nieces and nephew, and one of the nicest guys I have ever known. He reminded me a lot of Steve: patient, strong yet gentle, slow to anger and quick to help.

This morning, he called Susie to tell her he was going to be talking to her Grandmother, his mother, and that's where he decided to go, too. I believe that's what he is doing right now. A great reunion is taking place.

My heart is aching for Susie. Tomorrow morning, Susie and I will be driving to Montreal to be with her family. A service to honor Daniel will be held on December 20. Noah has some medical testing on Monday, after which he will join us in Canada.

I know God is good all the time, but right now I am having a hard time trying to come up with things that have been good in 2009. This year has been incredibly tough. Noah and Susie have lost both of their dads within nine months.

When Jesus got word that his dear friend died, he made the long walk to the man's tomb. Mary and Martha grieving and crying, and their friends cried with them. Among those crying was Jesus. He knows the pain of losing someone close, someone for whom he cared deeply. Jesus understands mourning. He understands grief. He didn't just tell Mary and Martha to "get over it" or "move on," but He cried with them and shared their loss.

Right now, as Jesus rejoices with Daniel in Heaven, He is grieving with us here. I will miss you Daniel. Thanks for being such a great dad to Susie and to Noah. I will never forget your smile.

God is good, all the time.

December 9, 2009

Noah arrived safely in Montreal yesterday afternoon, not feeling any better than he has. The test results have all come back alright, so we are waiting on the doctor to decide the next step.

Meanwhile, Susie's mom and grandma will do their best to help him put some weight back on. A nice diet of Poutine (French fries drizzled in brown gravy with cheese curds, a French Canadian treat) and French pastries should do the trick. My daughter-in-law is grieving her father, but she's still our ever strong Susie. She is the rock in her family, working hard to make sure that everything is done right and in a timely way.

There's an interesting story behind Daniel's funeral. About a year ago, there was a big strike in the funeral home business here in Montreal. During the strike, bodies were piling up. The system keeping track of identities began to disintegrate. There was a family who had a funeral and burial. One month later, they received a phone call asking when they were planning on burying the body. The first body they buried ended up being the wrong one. The same thing happened with a family who had taken home the ashes of a loved one, only to find out a couple of months later there was a stranger in their urn. Several other similar stories also came out of the strike.

Since the system was broken not too long ago, the funeral home has some requirements that seem strange but are apparently necessary. On Saturday, Daniel's body was taken from his home by ambulance to the hospital. He was pronounced dead and identified by his brother and son. They then moved him to the morgue where he was further identified by his wife, son and a couple of brothers.

On Monday, Daniel was moved from the morgue to the funeral home. When meeting with the funeral director, the family was informed that the body must be identified again by six to seven people. So today the funeral home will prepare the body for showing, put him in a suit and place him in a borrowed casket for one hour. The family has to be there from 7-8 p.m. to see him and sign some papers. After that the body will be transferred to where the cremation will take place, but it will be a minimum of four days before that process will happen.

The funeral will be held on Saturday, December 19. It will be a full day starting at eleven in the morning and with the actual service beginning at nine at night. I think that we will be returning to Grand Rapids within a day or two afterward.

Instead of flowers, Susie and her family would like people to donate money toward the Dominican vocational school project that Steve had been assisting with for years. The school is on the same grounds as the K-12 program where we have been serving since 1996. It now educates over 600 students every day, providing them with uniforms, books, health care, dental care and a way out of poverty. The vocational school is the next step in helping kids learn a skill, giving them the necessary tools to be employed, run a small business, make money and feed their families. Currently, the students at the vocational school learn computers, hair dressing, English, business training and electrical work. The missing element is auto repair. In a country of eight million people, with many, many vehicles but not much in the way of training on how to fix them, learning auto repair is a certain way to move out of destitution into a life of hope.

Steve was working with Cristian, our adopted son from the Dominican Republic, to make the dream of the vocational school a reality. Now the fulfillment of his dream is in sight. To finish the auto repair element, which includes purchasing the necessary tools, a crane to lift the engines, and books, will cost $14,200.

When the school is complete, there will be a dedication held to officially name it "The Steve Sorrelle Vocational School."

In the midst of sadness and death, God makes good things happen. Helping people in need, giving hope to the hopeless, bringing health to the sick and food to the hungry; those things are coming out of my family's losses.

God is good, all the time.

January 3, 2010

It is 2010. I made it. The holidays are over, my Christmas tree is neatly packed away, the refrigerator is completely devoid of champagne, and all the glitter is now inside the vacuum bag.

When I was celebrating Thanksgiving with my family in Connecticut, I didn't know if 2010 would ever arrive. I dreaded planning for the holidays without The Grinch (my favorite nickname for Steve and my favorite Dr. Seuss character).

We had our roles. He put up the tree. I decorated it. He brought the decorations up from the basement. I arranged them around the house. Together we would watch "It's a Wonderful Life" and "A Christmas Story." I would cry when Clarence got his wings, and he would laugh when Ralphy shot his eye out. I did the shopping, and he did the shoveling. Christmas morning, I would prepare quiche, monkey bread and sparkling grape juice, while he took a nap on the couch surrounded by gift wrapping, G.I. Joes, Nintendo games and Barbie dolls.

This was *our* Christmas story for twenty nine years.

This season, I was doing a pretty good job feeling sorry for myself. I had no desire to put up a Christmas tree. I did not want to go Christmas shopping, eat Christmas food, watch Christmas movies or go to Christmas parties. I did not want to have Christmas without Steve. I wanted to go far away and just skip December. I'm not sure I could have had a crappier year than 2009, but I was sure I just wanted it to be over.

Then my perspective changed. During the couple of weeks before Christmas when I would normally be decorating, baking, shopping, planning and watching sappy Lifetime movies, I was in Montreal grieving with Noah and Susie. I could no longer feel sorry for myself when my son and daughter-in-law were going through such an incredibly painful time.

While I was in Montreal, my dearest friends put up my Christmas tree and some other decorations. I had several people offer to shop for me. I even had invitations out for lunches and dinners.

Newly armed with a better attitude, I decided to embrace 2009 and count the blessings of the year:

I am so grateful I got to spend six weeks with Steve after he was diagnosed.

I am thankful my father, son and daughter made it possible for me to miss as much work as I needed to.

I am incredibly blessed to have been able to say "goodbye for now."

I have four of the greatest kids a mom could dream of having, and all three of my boys are married to truly wonderful women.

My grandbabies are a constant source of joy, and in July I get another one!

My best friend in high school continues to be the dearest friend now.

My relationship with my sister-in-law went from great to greater.

My health is much better now than it was a year ago, even with the little bout of strep throat I am experiencing right now.

I have incredible friends who love me.

I have family that supports and cares for me.

I have a roof over my head and food on the table.

In every area of my life I am blessed. From the people that I work with to the people I go to church with to my line dancing pals and my sweet neighbors, it's apparent God is really looking out for me in a big way.

Okay, so I didn't have anyone to kiss at midnight on New Year's Eve, but what I do have are people to hug me and love me despite my shortcomings (no height jokes, please).

I called Steve "Grinch" because he was so focused on the celebration of Christmas he did not get into the celebrating of "Christmas." While I was frantically trying to find just the right gifts, he was spending time in praise to God, Father of the Son, the Redeemer and Messiah. As I was wrapping, running, and wrestling the crowds, he was relaxed, refreshed and renewed in his faith.

But as he *Bah Humbug*-ed my ways, and I Grinched his, he never let me forget for one moment what the celebration is for, the birth of our Savior, Jesus Christ. Steve was my rock and my balance. He would rein me in when I would start to get out of control. He was my reality check.

Jesus, thanks for Steve. And thanks for the warning you gave me in a dream that he would be going "home" soon. Right after Steve's dad died, I dreamed that God told me Steve would be following him soon after, but everything would be alright. So I did have more than six weeks of warning. When all else fails, you are there.

I am ready to move, Lord. Please sell my house as quickly and painlessly as possible. I am getting pretty excited about that downtown condo living.

Love you, Lord. Please tell Steve "Happy New Year" for me. God is good, all the time.

January 4, 2010

I have been great at *making* New Year's resolutions for years. It's keeping them I have yet to master. But this is a new year, with new beginnings and new resolve.

First, I want to get off the self-pity, denial, and sad train I have been riding. I am putting it in writing so when I am celebrating the end of 2010, I can see I have accomplished what I set out to do:

1. **Get healthy!** I will try not to eat white things like sugar, flour, rice and potatoes, and I will exercise and fix my body. I have thrown away the cookies, tossed out the peanut brittle and disposed of the banana bread. Although, I might not exercise daily but several times each week or at least a couple. Line dancing does count as aerobics (or at least it should).

2. **Get connected!** I have survived breast cancer, but I haven't admitted to myself I was ever diseased. It still seems like an out of body experience. So many people have joined together to find cures and fight breast cancer, and without their efforts, I don't know where I would be today. I need to jump on that band wagon. In 2010 I will do at least one breast cancer walk, be available to people who have been diagnosed and get my tattoos finished.

3. **Get beyond the word "widow"!** My name is Kim Sorrelle, and I am a widow. There, I said it. I admit it. I am not the first and unfortunately will not be the last. I have snubbed my nose at books on grieving, passed on invitations to "sharing" groups, never stepped foot in Gilda's club and get angry every time a new Widowed Person's flyer arrived in the mail. How can I help anyone else get through this yuck if I keep paddling down the River of Denial? I resolve to put my oar in the other side of the canoe and take the right fork. I am going to attend a Griefshare group and figure out a way to help other women in similar circumstances.

4. **Get it done!** I am going to do whatever it takes to get the vocational school in Los Alcarizzos, Dominican Republic, finished. Steve and I worked in this very poor community for a number of years, trying to help kids find a way out of poverty. The vocational school compliments the K-12 Christian school which educates over 1000 students. The current offerings will be greatly enhanced by the addition of automobile

mechanics. I am determined to raise the remaining $14,000 to purchase the equipment, tools and space necessary to finish the project. On March 6, I will be hosting a fundraising event at English Hills, inviting "Home Party" consultants and non-profits like youth groups and sports teams to sell items giving a portion of the income toward the funds. I plan on going to the D.R. after the money is raised to attend the dedication of the Steve Sorrelle Vocational School.

5. **Get it down!** After much urging by several people, I am going to write a book.

6. **Get it right!** True friends give great advice. Loved ones try to help each other live better lives. Philosophers, poets and politicians are quoted and repeated, giving words of wisdom to the world. But to truly find words to live by, words that bring hope, words that build up, words that define, I turn to the Bible. Years ago Paul wrote to the people of Philippi, advising them on how to live: "Finally, brethren, whatever is true, whatever is honorable, whatever is right, whatever is pure, whatever is lovely, whatever is of good repute, if there is any excellence and if anything worthy of praise, dwell on these things. (Philippians 4:8, New American Standard Version.) This is my verse for 2010, great advice from a great advisor.

I will keep these resolutions. I will keep these resolutions. I will keep these resolutions.

So far, so good. Today I have only eaten a banana.

God is good, all the time.

February 7, 2010

Tomorrow will be eleven months since Steve died. Sometimes it seems like yesterday and sometimes it seems like it has been so long since I have seen him. If Steve walked through the door right now, somehow I would not be surprised. I would just get up, give him a big hug and ask him to take out the trash.

About a year ago, when Steve was in the hospital, a pastor from church came to visit. I remember asking him where the Bible states God will not give you more than you can handle. I had searched and come up empty. He told me that he didn't know, but knew it was there. I asked him to find it and let me know. I asked the hospital chaplain the same question. I asked every pastor, priest and rabbi I ran into, but never got an answer.

What I found in the Bible was just the opposite. When Paul wrote his second letter to the Corinthians, he said he was under pressure far beyond what he was able to endure. But that is where God stepped in, to carry Paul's burdens because he could not do it alone.

If God won't give you more than you can handle, I take that to mean that God gives you heartaches, disease, pain, conflict, war, earthquakes and tsunamis. I don't believe God gives us these things. I really believe these things happen because we live in a world with disease and death and disasters.

This morning my dear, sweet LeeAnne told me that Father Mark Przybysz addressed this very issue today at her church. I wish so badly I would have been there to hear him. He is a wonderful priest whom I greatly respect. Father Mark and I worship the same God, a God of peace, love, hope, joy and truth.

In Jeremiah 29:11, God says He knows the plans He has for us. They are plans to help us, not harm us, plans to give us hope and a future. God goes on to say that He will listen to us when we pray and if we look for Him we will find Him.

God has heard my prayers and yours as well. When Paul wrote about feeling like he was at the end of his rope, he knew God was there pulling him through, but he also knew the prayers of his friends were important. I like the way Eugene Peterson interprets Paul's words in "The Message":

"You and your prayers are part of the rescue operation — I don't want you in the dark about that either. I can see your faces even now, lifted in praise for God's deliverance of us, a rescue in which your prayers played such a crucial part."

Thank you for your prayers. When I think about how my life has changed in the last year, I cannot imagine arriving here alone. I am overwhelmed by the love, kindness and thoughtfulness that's been poured out to me. "Thank you" seems so insignificant. But I am truly grateful.

As far as my New Year's Resolutions go, I have eaten some white stuff but am back on track, will be walking in the Relay for Life in May, have checked the 'widow' box a few times on medical forms, and on March 6th, I am holding a fundraiser for the Steve Sorrelle Vocational School. I am working on "getting it right" and I am writing a book. In fact, I am writing two books.

I also started a blog on dating at forty eight. Oh my, it is crazy. I have decided to spend the next year "researching" on how to date since it has been a really long time. Find me at datingat48.wordpress.com. Read at your own risk.

God is good, all the time.

February 10, 2010

As far as my heath goes, I am doing alright. I did have a biopsy in January that showed some atypical cells. The biopsy was followed by a CAT scan, x-ray, tests on some bodily fluids, and waiting. So far, everything has come back pretty good. I do have a couple of kidney stones hanging around waiting to cause pain, but besides that I am A Okay. I will be having one other test on Friday and expect to get a clean bill of health.

It is February, *already*. That darn ground hog saw his shadow so I guess we will be having six more weeks of winter. Spring always seems to come at the same time every year so I am not sure why we rely on a little rodent to predict the calendar. Punxsutawney Phil *is* cute. I guess that is all that matters.

February also means Valentine's Day. I remember the first Valentine's Day with Steve. My expectations were huge. My dad and brothers had set the bar high. One year my brother bought his girlfriend (now wife) a box of chocolates. He opened the box and replaced a candy with a ring. Then he shrink wrapped the box so that it looked like it came right off the store shelf and had never been opened. I don't recall exactly what happened when my sister-in-law opened the box but I am sure she was pretty thrilled.

My dad always spoiled my mom with the biggest, most beautiful, heart-shaped box of chocolates he could find, complete with a sappy card and a dozen red roses. He would walk in the door after work with his arms full of treasures. There would be a little bit of hugging and kissing, and that's as far as I want to know. Every year romance was in the air; my brothers treated their girlfriends like queens and my mom always got the biggest gifts of all.

I remember how the day dragged on as I sat at my desk, trying to focus on work, but daydreaming instead about how my fiancé, Steve, would sweep me off my feet on our first Valentine's Day.

Giddy with excitement, I spent my lunch hour shopping in downtown Sparta buying him a sweater, candy and a card. *Oh, the anticipation was killing me. What would Steve do? Would he try to hide jewelry? Would it be a ring or a necklace or earrings? I was as excited to wear whatever it was to work the next day as I was to actually receive the precious gems. Certainly Steve had thought long and hard about the special holiday of love, preparing for days, maybe even weeks, ahead of time. I could just picture him in the Hallmark store reading each card carefully until he found just the right poem to express his nearly indescribable love for me. And the gift! How he must have agonized over finding the perfect present that would require no words, no special wrapping because of its utter transcendence. And one day, I would re-gift the prize to my daughter—perhaps on her wedding day!—telling of her father's incredible flair for romance, re-enacting the moment from our very first Valentine's Day when Steve surprised me beyond my wildest expectations!

When I arrived home from work, I saw Steve's baby blue Volkswagen Beetle already in the driveway. Running from the car, I reached for the front door knob only to have it opened before I could touch it. There was Steve, that gorgeous man, that hopeless romantic, waiting for me, opening the door for me, greeting me with his generous smile.

In his hands were the gifts which he extended with a smile. He gave me a small, heart-shaped, box of chocolates and three red roses.

Seriously, barely a handful of cheap chocolates and three grocery store flowers? Yes, that was it, the extent of his wildly romantic gift. There was nothing more, nothing hiding, nothing waiting, nothing else.

Who *was* this guy? I wondered what I was thinking. Was I really going to spend the rest of my life with a man who has no idea what to buy me for Valentine's Day? I questioned my sanity. This was the barometer against which all future Valentine's Days would be measured. The most romantic day of the year and he failed.

Steve had no idea why I would be disappointed. After all, he not only bought candy, but flowers too. And he did spend a good amount of time in the card aisle at the grocery store. It was one stop shopping, quick in and out. You see, Steve wanted to beat me to my house so he could be there waiting, at the door, for his Valentine. He had no idea I would be buying him gifts. Steve thought this was a day where the man brought the woman special treats but certainly did not expect anything in return. He loved the sweater, not because of the color or style but because it was the first Valentine's gift he had ever received, and from his love. And candy, his favorite, sea foam. The card was so sweet; the poem perfect. Oh, how he loved the gifts because they were from me. Meanwhile, I was totally discontent with my gifts.

Obviously, this was an issue that was going to have to be addressed. During our first year of marriage, Steve decided it was time for a heart to heart. What he viewed as a conversation, I remember as one of the best lectures I had ever received. Steve informed me that it was not him doing things wrong necessarily, but my expectations that came between us.

I found out then that Steve was not a mind reader. He did not know what I expected. He had no idea how *much* I expected.

I realized it was my expectations that started a lot of our fights early in our marriage.

I began to look at things much differently. I threw my expectations out the window. I realized I liked to cook for Steve, not for the praise, but because I loved him. I liked to live in a clean home. Writing "Kim hearts Steve" in the dust on the coffee table, then wiping it away with a Pledge covered cloth, making the cool lines in the shag carpet so that the fibers all stood at attention, and finding enough change for pizza night in the couch were all enjoyable acts to me.

Our marriage changed. Our relationship got so much better when I allowed Steve to be Steve and tell me nice things and do nice things for me in his way, not based on my expectations but because he loved me.

Sometimes I have made the same mistake with God. I expect Him to heal me when I am sick, heal Steve, heal everyone I know. I expect Him to provide for me a certain way. I expect Him to show Himself to people that do not believe in Him. I expect Him to do things my way because I know that it is the best way. But somehow, when I let God be God, He far exceeds my expectations.

God is good, all the time

February 21, 2010

I have some incredible friends who lost their twenty two-year-old daughter in a car accident today. She was a beautiful girl I coached for a little while. Her brother has been one of Noah's best friends for years (he also married a beautiful girl whom he met at our house).

I begged her to play volleyball, not just because she was a great athlete, but because I loved her spitfire attitude. Her family was the kind that gave much more than they received, and sacrificed well beyond any expectations. They really have hearts of pure gold. My heart aches for them today.

I wonder what it would be like to die as a child, to be swept off to the greatest playground in God's creation, with unending fruit snacks, Christmas every day and no more vaccinations. Heaven for children is, I think, living in a place that rolls up Willie Wonka's Chocolate Factory, Disney World, FAO Schwarz, and grandma's lap in one.

Heaven is incredible for the child, but their going to Heaven is horrible for the family and friends, and especially for the parents. That child would never know that for years to come, their loved ones on earth would think about what could have been. Every soccer game, birthday party, graduation, and wedding would be a partly painful occasion to imagine the child playing, celebrating, and coming down the aisle dressed in white.

The hole in the parents' hearts that only their child could fill might eventually diminish but it would never go away. In the innocence of childhood, with unquestioning faith, and the blessing of ignorance, the child would enjoy the absolute pleasures of paradise with contentment in knowing Mom and Dad would also be there shortly.

I am glad I didn't die when I was twenty two, as I was just beginning to realize I was not the center of the universe. As a new wife and mother, I was probably making more bad choices than good. Between my immaturity, lack of life skills and rebelliousness towards authority, I'm sure I offended more people than I helped.

I hope I don't die at 48. I am just beginning to grasp life. As I try to gain understanding, I realize now that I know so little. No longer the idealistic twenty two year old, but still, not so jaded by the twenty six extra years of disappointments and frustrations, I know I can make a difference.

I no longer aspire to change the entire world, but I know I can bring change, one life at a time. I have too much work to do. I am at my prime. My kids are all taking care of themselves, and I cook and do laundry for one.

Now, at forty eight, I have the time, passion and freedom to pursue my dreams. Relying more on God, trying to figure out how to love Him and please Him completely, living each day as it comes, I am working on listening more than talking, understanding more than arguing, and sacrificing more than indulging.

Before I become incorrigible, incontinent and insane, I want to quietly go in my sleep, while hearing voices of loved ones saying "she lived a full life." I want to hear "She was a woman with great faith" echo off the church rafters at my funeral, and I want to hear "Well done" from my Father.

God is good, all the time.

March 19, 2010

March 8th marked the anniversary of Steve's last breath here and his first breath in Heaven. He made it! And so did I.

Upon discovering I was still in my pajamas at 2:00 p.m. that afternoon, my daughter-in-law, Laci, called her mom. By 2:30

p.m., my dear friend Tami was at my door with a smile, a huge bouquet of gorgeous yellow roses, and a shoulder to cry on.

It's funny how some days, dates, and moments sucker punch me. Instead of being my usual optimistic, ambitious, grab-the-tiger-by-the-tail self, I turn into a pathetic slug that desires nothing more than elastic waist sweat pants, potato chips, chocolate and "The Price Is Right." Then I look at a calendar and realize it is the anniversary of our first kiss, Steve's birthday or the 8th of the month.

Michigan weather has been beautiful for the past few days. The sun is shining and it smells like spring time. The outside is so inviting, with no jacket required. But the bearer-of-bad-news meteorologist predicts snow for tomorrow.

It's a case of weather imitating life. With a lilt in your step, a twinkle in your eye and a whistle on your lips, you step off the curb and get hit by a Mack truck. Sometimes life is like that.

Finding joy in the sunny days is easy. But on the dark days, joy can be buried under the snow. Sometimes there's little room for happiness when it is hard to see the sun through the clouds. So much time can be lost worrying about the tough days instead of enjoying the blissful ones.

Ezra and Nehemiah told people who were hearing the words of the Bible for the first time not to mourn because the joy of the Lord is their strength.

When we are weak, He gives us strength. When we are sad, He gives us joy. When we are down, He throws us a rope.

The tough days will happen, but when they do I am going to allow God to bring me joy in the middle of my sadness. Will you? We can live in such fear of a rotten peanut, we don't enjoy the hundreds of good salty, tasty treats in the bag.

Okay. So I did not want to get out of bed on the 8th. But God's joy can still overwhelm me sometimes. Aurora's jokes can make me laugh. My friends bring out the best in me. And roses are my favorite flowers.

I would rather be happy than sad, laugh than cry, smile than scowl. The glass is half full. My friend, enjoy the good things in life without fear that the tables will turn.

In Psalms, it is written that crying might last for the night but joy comes in the morning. The sentence just before tells that God might get angry once in a while, but His love and His favor wrap across a lifetime.

Tomorrow morning I leave for Haiti. Since the earthquake, I have been living and breathing and existing to help the people of Haiti. Working with my good friend, Doug Porritt, at Rays of Hope for Haiti, we have sent over 250,000 pounds of food, water and medical supplies with more being sent out from our warehouse weekly. I am going down to connect with our Haitian partners to see what more we can do. Please keep me in your prayers.

God is good, all the time.

Epilogue

A lot has happened in the last year and three quarters.

In July of 2010, Paul and Laci welcomed their first child, a beautiful boy, and named him Stephen Paul. I cannot think of a more wonderful tribute to Paul's dad, my hubby. Stephen is, of course, flawless. He has brown curly hair and his dad's hazel eyes. He is smart and handsome and funny and the sweetest little bundle in the world.

Now in 2011 two more grandbabies have been born. Scarlett Mae, Stephen's little sister, and William Franklin, boy number three for Cristian and Sarah. Both are healthy, precious and wonderful.

Noah and Susie graduated from Western Michigan University, Noah with a degree in Micro Biology and Susie in Criminal Justice. Yellow cords at graduation indicated Summa Cum Laude and Magna Cum Laude, with Susie just ahead of Noah (go Susie! Go Noah!). Noah also had red, white and blue cords signifying his U.S. Military Veteran status. This gained him a loud ovation. Steve would have been so proud. So would've Daniel. So would've my mom.

Noah has applied for graduate school and is waiting for acceptance. Meanwhile he is working in a research lab and hopes to be published soon. Susie is waiting to see where Noah is going to be enrolled so that she knows where to apply. Meanwhile she is working retail and keeping Noah in line.

Amanda got married! She is in love with Ray. Ray is very sweet to her and the girls. Aurora is now in first grade and

Cordelia is in pre-school. The last time I came home from Haiti, Aurora informed me that she will be saving her money so she can help the poor kids too. Cordie has yet to learn how to walk, she continues to flit, float and dance from place to place. I pray that she dances for the rest of her life. Walking is for the ordinary. Dancing is for Cordelia.

Luke is out of the Navy. He and Megan are both going to college, Luke for electrical engineering and Megan for teaching. Crichton had his school Christmas program and sang his little heart out in a way that only Crichton can. Evayah is growing up quickly and wants to be just like her cousin Aurora. I had the opportunity to live with Luke, Meg, Crichton and Evayah for nine months after Luke's discharge. The kids think I tell the best stories ever, but their parents think that I am a little crazy. I think the kids are right.

Paul is running the family businesses and doing an outstanding job. Laci is taking great care of Stephen and Scarlett and Paul.

Cristian and Sarah are flying back and forth from Michigan to the Dominican Republic. The vocational school is thriving, and everyone who graduates finds employment. Leo, C.J. and William are three peas in a pod, bi-lingual, early talkers, early walkers, early everything, sweet, precious boys.

As for me, I recently turned into Mary Richards of the Mary Tyler Moore show—I can turn the world on with my smile (maybe). I sold my house in the suburbs and had two weeks to pack up a lifetime. I found a great little condo in a downtown high rise. I don't have to unfold a sofa bed each night but I can vacuum my entire new place in about ten minutes flat. Just like Miss Richards I rarely date, love the people that I work with, and have spunk. And although Mr. Grant hates spunk, I still expect him to walk through the door any moment and give me some straight-to-the-point fatherly advice.

Traveling to Haiti has become a habit as Executive Director of Rays of Hope for Haiti. Since my visit in March of 2010, I have returned to Haiti fifteen times. I am Haitian now, except when I am American.

I am a widow. I have embraced it. Widow has joined other descriptive words like mom, Uma, daughter, short, funny (in a good way), etc. There are statistics related to widows just like everything else it seems. Most widows change churches, lose most of their friends, have major financial problems and gain twenty pounds. Even though I try hard to not fit the mold, I did just change churches, but I hope that I didn't lose any friends, and praise God my finances are surviving. As for the twenty pounds, it comes and goes.

Life. I don't know how things happen so quickly. One day I am a carefree ten-year-old playing kick ball in a neighbor's back yard, and the next I am an Uma to nine little ones. One day I am walking down the aisle holding onto my dad's arm with the man of my dreams waiting for me by the altar, and the next I am holding on to nearly thirty years of memories. One day I am mowing the acre lawn surrounding the home where my family had last lived all together and the next I am living in a high rise condo building downtown.

I love my life. I am truly blessed with family, friends and fun. I love my job, my new place and my haircut. I love being an Uma, a humanitarian and a friend. I love summer, spring and fall (winter is a bit cold for me!). I love Jesus, the creator of all things, the rock, the healer, the restorer, the one I lean on. I love

Steve and miss him so much. Sometimes I cry but most of the time I smile at the memories.

As the Paul Williams song says, "How will you make it on your own? ... Girl this time you're all alone."

I'm going to make it after all.

God is good, all the time.

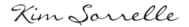

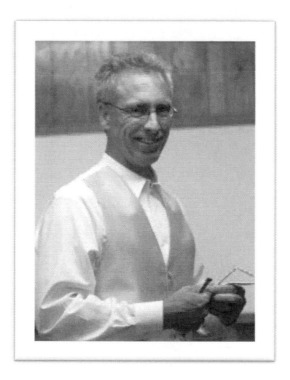

Steve Sorrelle at Paul and Laci's wedding, July, 2008

Donations in Steve Sorrelle's honor may be given to Rays of Hope for Haiti to help continue the work in a community of nearly 300,000 people in the Dominican Republic. Currently, there is a K-12 School with over 1,000 students, Vocational School, Water Purification System, Community Development and a Home Building Project.
Send donations to: Rays of Hope for Haiti
446 Grandville Ave. SW
Grand Rapids, MI 49503.